MY
THIRD
LIFE

Multiple Sclerosis hit me.
But I hit back!

ROLAND TASSLER

TABLE OF CONTENTS

So much talk, so little empathy
Increasing reduction
A glimmer of hope, then disappointment
Down again
Just one way out

CHAPTER 3: THE START OF MY THIRD LIFE

The year 2014
My friend the diary
Why do handcraft despite the handicaps?
My hunger for knowledge
Where does the fight for health start?
Our thoughts are the key – but only the right ones!

CHAPTER 4: MY PHYSICAL CONDITION IN JANUARY 2014

CHAPTER 5: THE NECESSARY MOTIVATION AND GOALS

Give yourself a chance
First: focus on success by setting realistic daily goals
Bigger goals
My '5-S' Strategy for self-motivation
Creating the right dream
Second: I had to lose weight
Third: Learning to move properly
How to get healthy again?

CHAPTER 6: HELPFUL NUTRITION

About good health and bad health, food for life or pleasure
Alkaline or acidic
What helped me

CHAPTER 7: VITAMIN D3 – THE SUN HORMONE!

Vitamin D3 – the 'mains switch' of our body's functions
The sun as a vitamin D3 source
How I came to high concentrate dosages of vitamin D3

CHAPTER 8: THE MOST IMPORTANT THING OF ALL IS WATER!

Drinking water heals – without water nothing is possible!
A word on fungi in the body

CHAPTER 9: ELIMINATION AND DETOXIFICATION

The intestines and our health
I need a target, and the will to make a change
The skin as excretory organ
Scrutinizing the relationships in our body
The kidneys and their limits
Beyond the lungs
Nutrition and detox - a conclusion

CHAPTER 10: OUT THOUGHTS

Thoughts are life-determining!
Are we able to change ourselves?
How does our environment shape our thoughts and behaviour?
How you can change your thinking and your behaviour

CHAPTER 11: DEATH AND IMMORTAL LIFE

The fear of dying and getting healthy
Our birth came with an expiry date
We all are made of cosmic atoms
Consciousness energy
What comes after death?
Living in the present

CHAPTER 12: THE DVD WHICH CHANGED MY LIFE

The first meeting
Vitamin D3 - first drops
About my diary records

CHAPTER 13: EXTRACTS FROM MY DIARY

Diary entries

CHAPTER 14: WHAT HAS CHANGED IN MY LIFE?

CHAPTER 15: WHAT ARE THE NEXT STEPS?

My second book: Masterplan zum Erfolg (Masterplan for Success)
My third book: Angst im Kopf (A Psyche of Fear)
My fourth book: Tabu (Taboos)
My fifth book: Mein Freund Gott (My friend god)
What I do today
Where to find me

FORWARD

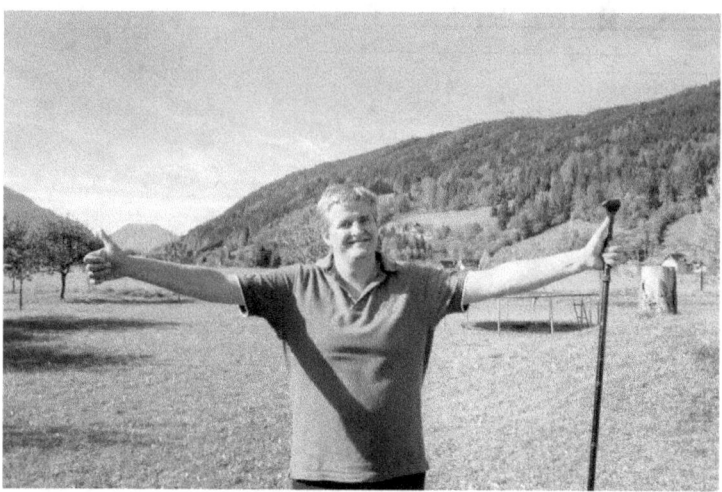

My name is **Roland Tassler**. I was born in Vienna, Austria, in 1967. At the time of writing this book I was 49 years old, and have suffered with the continual/chronic degenerative form of the autoimmune illness *Multiple Sclerosis (MS)* since 2003.

I would like to say from the start that I write as I speak, and my style may therefore appear somewhat strange at first. This is simply how I am; I never learnt how to write a book and I had never planned to write one. However, under the circumstances, I feel the need to write everything down before I forget it. And due to the physical limitations of my illness this book was typed with 2 fingers on my notebook. My grammar may not be the best and I ask you to kindly indulge me my errors. I believe that you, my readers, will be able to grasp the essential content despite the errors, and if you find any mistakes please feel free to keep them!

As I am neither a doctor nor a medical expert I am not allowed to use terms such as 'healing', or make recommendations to the reader in one way or another. I speak purely from personal experience with my own body. Any claims recommendations for particular therapies would also be illegal. I have therefore only written about my own personal experiences and sincerely encourage each individual to search for and try out their own solutions. The road to health is a continual, transformative and dynamic process and must be checked at every stage. One needs to observe closely and be ready to change at any stage.

Should someone simply copy something from my story they may well have a completely different result. It must be emphasised here that my 'personal therapy' has been developed specifically for my own body. At the outset I weighed 110 kg and the prerequisites and conditions are naturally quite different to someone weighing 60 kg. Therefore please note that what I share in this book is based on my own personal condition and experiences.

There were two reasons for writing this book: The first was to give hope to those who feel hopeless. I know how empty life can be without hope. I am just like you – not a therapist who hasn't had any personal experience himself. I would particularly like to share my experiences of the last 2 years since they changed my life. Such a marked physical improvement in such a short time should not be kept to oneself. There IS hope, and indeed for everyone!

The second reason for writing this book is to draw attention to the possibility of healing oneself, or at least changing ones condition significantly through less conventional medicines and therapies.

I am no medical expert but I have something even better: I have experience with my own body. And that makes a big difference, as I explain later.

This book aims therefore to help by offering other points of view when it comes to the concepts 'incurable' or 'terminal' or 'chronic'. It shows new ways out of apparently insolvable, hopeless situations. With this book you will hopefully find a way to create more joy and energy for yourself and find new impulses towards a healthy life.

This is the RIGHT book for you, if….

- you are stuck in a hopeless life crisis
- you suffer from Multiple Sclerosis or any other incurable disease without prospects for the future
- you are prepared to take your life into your own hands

This is NOT the right book for you, if…

- you already know everything and don't need any advice
- you completely trust conventional medicine and see no need for alternatives
- you leave your wellbeing up to others

As a **bonus** I have included a list of internet websites at the end of the book. There you will find short videos of actual places and events as described in this book.

I have also added my daily program along with a list of important internet links and a list of books and other resources that could help you reach your goal, whether you have MS or not.

This is my story of how I went from being a bedridden invalid to being without a wheelchair and even driving a car. In this book I show how I achieved it, and how *everyone* can. I want to give hope to all those suffering from hopeless and incurable diseases. You are not alone with your worries and fears. We can often achieve significantly more than what others may have us believe, including conventional specialists. There is always a solution, somewhere. We must just look for it. It's worth it.

Roland Tassler, Vienna Austria, 1 May 2016

CHAPTER 1: THE CIRCUMSTANCES AROUND MS – CONDITIONS AND NORMS

The MS health environment

To help you understand my situation better I would like to describe my illness (MS) in the context of my personal 'health' environment and how this influenced me. In later chapters I will explain how my illness at first controlled and degraded me, and how everyone around me regarded this helpless condition as normal and unavoidable to the point of even supporting this sentiment.

I will give you insights into how I was able to overcome these major obstacles. Many things happened that resulted in a change in my basic beliefs; how I viewed my illness and the chances of healing myself, and which helped me to resume the responsibility for myself which I had long given up.

I would like to start by describing the health environment because it denied me the idea of considering alternative effective options.

The system of conventional medicine

Academic medicine should by all accounts be there for the good of the patient. The question is if it really does achieve this, or if it is a tool of or in cohorts with the powerful pharmaceutical industry? Are doctors encouraged to be there for their patients or to earn as much money as possible? Is a doctor allowed to concern himself with the healing and sustainable health of his patients, or does he merely make the symptoms of the suffering easier to bear? Essentially, the latter is not what 'healing' is.

It would appear that the medical system as it currently is, is based on a business model which focuses more on profits than less expensive and more effective cures from natural remedies.

This leads one to further question if the pharma industry is more interested in those 'regular'/'chronic' patients who keep them going. True? That is exactly how things function in any system where money will flow so long as people remain ill. A sick person is the best customer because one doesn't earn anything from healthy people.

Do universities only acknowledge medical students who do verbatim what the professor tells them to do? What happens when he starts to think independently and raises critical questions when noticing that it's not the humanitarian element of the doctor, rather the business model (at the cost of the patient or the medical aid) that becomes the primary focus? He may well have problems with his grades and reputation down the line.

Could doctors gradually 'unlearn' to heal patients while their earnings increase steadily through their chronically ill patients? Once, at one lecture, a lady representing the doctors admitted that, "Doctors also need to earn a living from something!" Of course they do! That is quite understandable. But my question is "Why don't doctors heal when they can and should be able to?" Everyone can draw his own conclusions.

I certainly don't want to suggest that all doctors practice like that. No, there are also many 'moral' and good doctors. Doctors contracted into medical aids are under a lot of pressure which is why they do what they do.

Perhaps they see no alternative. Perhaps they don't even notice it any more. Private doctors, in comparison, don't have such pressure and can therefore give their patients much more time. The hook is that you have to be able to afford them. Think about it: to which doctor would you go if money wasn't an issue? Exactly! Could there perhaps be two 'classes' of doctors?

Medicine vs. science

Why does conventional medicine lag so many years behind scientific research? Are certain discoveries being covered up or held back from it? Or do they deny 'inconvenient' findings where healthier options may result in decreased profits? This assumption becomes ever clearer. My stomach turns when I think of it. How does one explain to a dying cancer patient that a particular medicine that could possibly save him is prevented by law as it could have side effects? I could image the cancer patient has bigger worries than 'side effects' when comes to his life. I am not speaking about medication such as Contergan, known as thalidomide, the administering of which had nothing to do with a life and death illness. I am speaking about medication that could actually help but which is withheld from the market for economic reasons.

Scientific research on MS

There are currently several researches being done on MS that demonstrate how it can be overcome, or at least significantly improved. Various options are indicated e.g. where vitamin B treatment on MS patients was positively received and showed outstanding success.

The Tecfidera Preparation, which was initially recommended by medial aids for psoriasis, is known to have helped MS patients.

As soon as the pharmaceutical industry noticed how effective it was for MS, the price was increased beyond the reach of the average patient. The cost of a year's supply went from USD 2000- to USD 55 000-. Please read:http://www.srf.ch/konsum/themen/gesundheit/gierige -pharmafirma-so-zockt-sie-schwerkranke-ab

Also worth a mention are the vitamin D3 and stem cell treatments. But as long as the results don't make economic sense to the 'system' the solutions remain out of reach. It is that simple.

My road is just one of many but it is accessible and doable even for those who do not have big budgets. This road is built on taking responsibility for oneself, and it shows that one can achieve a lot after doctors have given up.

What is MS actually?

To clarify: MS is not the same as Amyotrophia Lateral Schlerosis (known as ALS).

MS is described in Wikipedia [23.10.2016] as follows:

'Multiple sclerosis (MS) is a demyelinating disease in which the insulating covers of nerve cells in the brain and spinal cord are damaged. This damage disrupts the ability of parts of the nervous system to communicate, resulting in a range of signs and symptoms, including physical, mental, and sometimes psychiatric problems.

Specific symptoms can include double vision, blindness in one eye, muscle weakness, trouble with sensation, or trouble with coordination.

MS takes several forms, with new symptoms either occurring in isolated attacks (relapsing forms) or building up over time (progressive forms). Between attacks, symptoms may disappear completely; however, permanent neurological problems often remain, especially as the disease advances.

While the cause is not clear, the underlying mechanism is thought to be either destruction by the immune system or failure of the myelin-producing cells. Proposed causes for this include genetics and environmental factors such as being triggered by a viral infection. MS is usually diagnosed based on the presenting signs and symptoms and the results of supporting medical tests.

There is no known cure for multiple sclerosis. Treatments attempt to improve function after an attack and prevent new attacks. Medications used to treat MS, while modestly effective, can have side effects and be poorly tolerated. Physical therapy can help with people's ability to function. Many people pursue alternative treatments, despite a lack of evidence. The long-term outcome is difficult to predict, with good outcomes more often seen in women, those who develop the disease early in life, those with a relapsing course, and those who initially experienced few attacks. Life expectancy is on average 5 to 10 years lower than that of an unaffected population.

Multiple sclerosis is the most common autoimmune disorder affecting the central nervous system. In 2013, about 2.3 million people were affected globally with rates varying widely in different regions and among different populations. That year about 20,000 people died from MS, up from 12,000 in 1990.

*The disease usually begins between the ages of 20 and 50
and is twice as common in women as in men.
MS was first described in 1868 by Jean-Martin Charcot.
The name multiple sclerosis refers to the numerous scars
(sclerae—better known as plaques or lesions) that develop
on the white matter of the brain and spinal cord. A number
of new treatments and diagnostic methods are under
development.'*

Herewith a summary of the most important symptoms of
this illness:

- chronic inflammation and damaging of the outer
  layer of the nerves
- the whole nervous system is affected by it
- it can show itself in any of the neurological
  symptoms where pain, discomfort and restrictions
  arise at any stage anywhere in the body
- the cause is still not clear
- the illness is not curable

The Sword of Damocles and the freedom of choice to decide

I feel like the legendary Damocles of olden times,
where MS is the sword that hung over me. As with
Damocles, I had the choice of taking my place at the
king's table (in terms of the limited choice offered by
conventional medicine) over which the sword hung.

Many people do not recognise the variety of options
when it comes to making choices for their own personal
health. This is the reason that I am writing this book and
why I give public lectures. I want to open your eyes to the
range of possibilities when making decisions about your
health.

CHAPTER 2: MY SECOND LIFE...

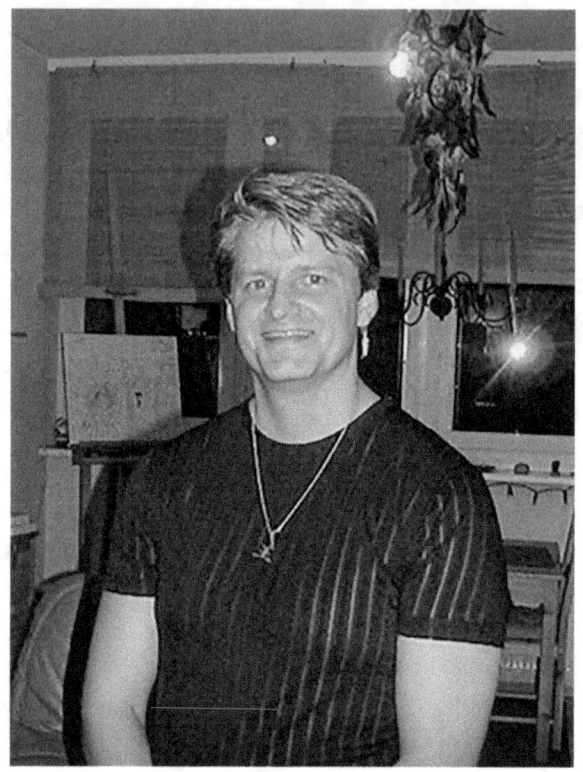

My 'first life' was the life prior to the illness. I was actually pretty happy with that life!

My 'second life' was the one with the illness. I would happily spare you this story but it would be good to understand how such an illness can affect an independent person. The early stages are different for everyone.

The progress of the illness is also dependent on how each individual deals with it. In this chapter I will briefly describe how this illness burdened me over the years.

My 'third life' started when I decided to bring my MS under control, which took me on a path of significant improvements and life-changes that continue to this day.

This is my story. At the end of the book there is a photo gallery where you can see my progress.

My first life – before I became ill

Before I became ill I was very athletic; I went jogging, I went to the fitness centre, and I joined various Boogie Woogie dance courses. Aside from having had the common flu a few times I had never been seriously ill. *See picture one in the gallery.*

My second life – with the illness

The first sign of MS was my inability to **sleep through the night** with the age of 35. I would fall asleep in the evening and after two or three hours I would wake up as if someone had pushed a button. Then I would not be able to fall asleep again. During the day I would be tired which eventually led to me being stressed, and it had a negative impact on my performance at work.

I also had recurring **dizzy spells** which were often so bad that I would fall against walls or door frames. It was like being inebriated while actually being sober.

The dizziness would come suddenly and sometimes last for hours, or even days and weeks. The longest phase was three weeks in a row! I would often get so dizzy that I felt nauseous if I closed my eyes.

Falling asleep was horrible. I had to put one leg on the floor outside the bed in order to help me keep my balance and feel stable.

Naturally I went to a doctor, but was constantly told that it came from tension in the neck area. So I went to physiotherapy and was massaged and received treatment with electric currents. But the dizziness would return again and again.

One day, at my fitness centre, I noticed that my body was unusually **weak**. I was unable to lift the heavier weights that I had previously lifted without any problem. They felt heavier than usual and I couldn't do my normal number of reps. When a bar-bell fell out of my hand and hit me on the head I started wondering seriously if everything was OK with me.

I then began to notice that my legs would tremble badly after training and that the **recovery period** after each session was **unusually long**. From experience I knew I could expect to exercise the same muscles again after two days, but suddenly I needed a week or more before I could use the same muscles again. Eventually I had to stop training with weights altogether.

The deterioration

The **muscular pains** started soon thereafter, which led to **chronical nerve inflammation**. That was even worse. My skin and certain muscles became so inflamed and sensitive to even the slightest touch, that getting dressed or covering myself with a blanket at night was impossible.

At this stage I could hardly think about sleeping with or dating anyone. If I fell asleep it was due to **overtiredness** and **exhaustion**. My body just shut down for a short time. I had heard about similar symptoms from training buddies who were treating themselves with various 'medications' designed for bodybuilding, but that couldn't have applied to me as I never played with any dangerous enhancement or stimulant drugs.

Unbearable pains in my **hips**, my **right elbow** and both my **wrists** followed. I could no longer think about training or dancing.

Two months later **sensory disturbances** appeared in the **fingers** of my right hand and in my right **upper arm**. These appeared as numbness, itching and extreme sensitivity to **temperature changes**.

Washing myself was like running the gauntlet. The water felt too hot on one area of my body but too cold on another, although this had less to do with the actual **temperature** of the water, it simply hurt. When taking a shower, for example, the water under my arms was too cold while on my legs it was too hot.

Times of **pain** alternated with pain-free time. The doctor said I should quit my training for a period of time and then I would be fine. According to him it all came from too much stress and exertion during training.

But the situation did not improve. **Muscle weakness, unsteady gait** and **coordination disorder** started to appear and sometimes I even needed a **walking aid**. My right leg eventually became completely stiff as **paralysis** spread over various muscles. My left leg wasn't affected as much but even there I had certain ailments such as **skin irritations**. In the beginning some of the **MS attacks** were so severe that I would be bedridden for weeks.

All this took place over the first five years. During this time there were constant visits to the doctor and I was often told directly or indirectly that I was moaning for nothing and I was even called a hypochondriac. But I knew that there was something wrong with me.

Being **fatigued** immediately after only a couple of minutes of effort, and having **exhaustion** lasting for hours, were also symptoms. But what bothered me the most was the chronic tiredness and **giddiness** which meant I would often fall, which was very dangerous.

In addition I was **temperature sensitive**. In summer I was forced to stay in my flat with the doors and windows closed and the air conditioner running 16 hours a day.

There were times when I wasn't able to leave my flat for weeks. A temperature of 77° Fahrenheit was excruciating as it felt like 104° for me.

My central nervous system affected various areas. Already, at an early stage of my illness, I suffered from a **weak pelvic floor**. That meant that I no longer had any control over my bladder or bowels. A walk to the toilet became an important event in my life. I drove, so to speak, from toilet to toilet. Alternatively I could have chosen to wear a diaper or stay home the whole time. I hit rock bottom in my life. At least this is what I thought. But as it turned out, it wouldn't be the last time.

Finally the diagnosis!
I went from physician to physician but none of them were able to tell me why my health was so rapidly deteriorating. I had never had problems with my eyes but now I was seeing 'diplopic' (double) images' - a typical symptom of MS. But it took five years and a lot of investigation until I finally got the diagnosis. **Multiple Sclerosis (MS).** This happened at Christmas 2008. It was the second 'incurable' disease in my life. The first one was psoriasis from which I had suffered for years. At this stage I didn't even know what MS was. I went to the AKH (the General Hospital in Vienna) several times to try and get some answers about my physical condition, but in vain.

Classic MS therapy and the side effects

The doctors opted for the route of conventional medicine and prescribed a medication called Copaxone (Glatiramer acetate) which I injected for a month only early in 2009. Many MS patients are treated with this drug. But when I experienced the side effects I knew instinctively that I would have a much better life without this medication:

Up to now, therapies such as with Interferon beta usually focussed on repressing the immune attack against the myelin sheaths. But they have only a limited effect and to some degree cause severe side effects. Furthermore they serve to only decelerate the progress of the illness as they can't stop or reverse the process. [4] *(Original text only available in German)*

'Limited effect' was described by my then doctor as being effective in only 25 – 30 % of all cases! Well, this means that 70 – 75% of all MS patients are further damaged by the side effects of the drug. I thought to myself that doctors had all gone crazy, and left!

Statistical facts: deaths caused by the side effects of medication

Here comes the bombshell! Please note! The following numbers are a comparison between Austria and the USA. I found these figures in a calculation example on the internet. It did state that one can't compare Austria with the USA, but everyone is able to draw their own conclusions:

Heading: death caused by the side effects of medication

Source:
http://www.pressetext.com/news/19980417015www.press
etext.at/news/980417015/

USA

- Inhabitants: approx. 305 million
- Deaths due to medication per year: 100,000
- Represents: approx. 0.03 % of the population
- In comparison – soldiers who died in the Iraq war: approx. 4,000 (as at 25 March 2008)

Austria

- Inhabitants: approx. 8 million
- Deaths due to medication per year: 2,400
- Represents: approx. 0.03 % of the population
- In comparison:
  - **Road fatalities per year: approx. 880**, represents 0.01 % of the population
  - **Fatal accidents at work per year: approx. 192**, represents 0.003% of the population
  - **Deaths through drowning: approx. 112**
  - **Accidents caused by fire, flames: approx. 57**
  - **Accidents through falling: approx. 999**

o   **Accidents through poisoning: approx.**
160
o   **Total of deaths per year: approx. 2400,**
represents 0.03% of the population

The risk of dying from medication is therefore 2.7 times higher than dying from a fatal accident in road traffic!

To these figures one must still add deaths resulting from incorrect dosage of medication. I don't say you must stop taking medicine. I rather suggest you think twice before taking it! Of course medication is important and good, but one has to take responsibility for oneself and check out everything one does first.

Healers, gurus, quacks

With my statement above I don't mean to imply that I am against conventional medicine. It was simply not the right solution for me. At that stage I had to take responsibility for myself and starting looking at alternatives like TCM (Traditional Chinese Medicine) and homeopathy.

I would also like to state that by nature I am rather a realistic thinker, a sceptical half-believing person. Indeed I understand that there is more to life, but there are also a lot of self-proclaimed 'healers', 'gurus' and 'charlatans'. I suggest one be very careful before parting with money for such services. It is an unfortunate fact that a critically ill person can be very easily exploited financially.

Even I made the mistake of trying out some 'well known' healers. But their treatments were neither helpful nor harmful (except for my wallet). I was very vulnerable in this time of desperation and fear.

Shameless people promise you everything imaginable and you hold onto the prospect of a miracle healing, and continue to pay money into their bank accounts month after month. They brag about people they have allegedly healed, but you never get to meet these people. Even friends and relatives try to help by recommending some or other person who has already saved the lives of many sick people through his unique 'treatment'.

None of these were ever able to help me. And this included many 'well known healers'. One such healer, who lives in Brazil, charges nothing for the treatment itself but one has to pay for accommodation on his farm. Then there is the cost of the flight, and when adding it all up a six-month treatment can result in a very unpleasant surprise. In my experience such treatments don't work at all.

I know a young woman suffering from MS who flew to this 'healer' in Brazil. After six months she returned in a worse condition than before. Of course one has to pay for a real health counsellor too. If someone is able to give real and good advice which is actually helpful, he or she has to charge for their time and knowledge. No one should be expected to work free of charge. But all that should be within reasonable limits!

So- called 'gurus' and 'miracle healers' on the other hand, who make a living from your money from month to month, perhaps even over years, are simply cheaters in my opinion.

One also has to ask how long one can afford the therapy. There are therapies which are supposed to bring results after a long time period, but which are probably never going to work and are, of course, vehemently justified with a host of excuses. They are just a pure waste of money! Clearly, everyone would give the shirt off their back to get the 'miracle pill', but there is no such remedy.

What I do for my general health

The turn- around in my health took a very long time and cost a lot of money, but in a different way to what one might think. Sure one has to spend money on well-considered purchases too, which in any case everyone does. I began by buying better quality foods. Organic fruit and vegetables may cost a bit more but they pay off in the long term with improved physical health and a sense of wellness. I am not suggesting one should suddenly become an 'eco-guru', but it may help to start buying food in a more conscious way. Of course it needs to be affordable, and foods that I can afford to buy in a better quality I will certainly buy.

Nutrition as a solution

It is important to recognise that clean, healthy food is an essential element for good health. Regardless of how one lived previously, as soon as **you want** to change your state of health seriously, you have to be willing to step out of your comfort zone to some degree and reconsider your habits. Naturally you can ignore them and say, "Oh no, it's not so important..." But in the end it is your decision - it's about YOUR life and YOUR body. In my opinion moaning has never helped anyone. The type of life-style we have lived has brought us to where we are now. One needs to recognise when one is vulnerable, and accept that real change may be well be necessary, before something even worse may happen. And I am not referring to an accident!

A typical example is Diabetes Type 2. It is common knowledge that this form of diabetes is likely to occur through a continual bad diet and consumption of wrong foods. One can easily prevent Diabetes Type 2 at an early stage by changing the diet! Type 2 diabetes is insidious at the beginning and is therefore not always taken seriously. But in every case the impact is dramatic: Heart disease, heart attacks, strokes and even blindness are possible consequences. Even leg amputation or kidney failure.

British scientists have shown in a study that it is possible to heal Diabetes Type 2 through a selective diet. Who is responsible for the healing? The patient himself!

At this point I would like to add the point that the food industry, together with the advertising industry, contributes a great deal to the current negative health environment. Naturally it is up to everyone to buy the right foodstuffs, but when one takes a more precise look at the lobby which for decades, through various ads and campaigns, has tried to sell milk as the BEST food of all, or margarine, with claims that they are all healthy products, which is not only misleading but completely untrue, it makes it very difficult for one to decide what is really good and what isn't.

The healing process

Each body needs time to heal and get well, on a very individual basis. Each body is unique and therefore needs individual attention, but the basic steps of healing are similar with all of us. One very successful approach is to first detox the body, and then support its process of building up again. But this also costs money.

One needs a large dose of courage to dare to go in a new direction, while at the same time taking care of oneself each step of the way. I mean living with real 'self-responsibility', in other words, not believing everything the media tells us but rather to question things and inform yourself on how to deal with new, possibly unknown facts.

Doctors are not able to help you with MS. Even though they 'try' to help, they are not able to stop or reverse MS. The reason is not that doctors are incapable. Indeed they do try, but they can't really help you.

It's the same with most chronic illnesses. They are generally not able to do much more than 'make it bearable'.

Only you yourself are able to heal yourself, if you know how to, and if you want to. To claim here that one can heal or reverse every condition at any stage would also be wrong. One must also consider the extent of the damage or injuries which are caused by the medication and the illness itself.

Much more is possible than one imagines

I believe that we are capable of much more than we can ever imagine. I was a hopeless case according to the doctors. They had given up on me. But today I am able to walk. Who would have thought that someone suffering from MS, bedridden and condemned to a wheelchair, would be able to walk one day, alone?

For the doctors I was a hopeless case, but for me I wasn't a hopeless case and I reclaimed my responsibility for myself. Only then did logical thinking, study and hard work on myself follow. Help came only when I started looking for it, when I was inwardly ready to help myself. Help came in the form of people who supported me and gave me good and wise advice. So much is possible if one doesn't give up! The wise Goethe once wrote:

"Grey, dear friend, is all theory, but green is the life of the golden tree"
(My interpretation: Grey is the theory, what is important is the actual experience!)

So much talk, so little empathy

What does that mean? There are many people who have a lot to say about illnesses, but who have themselves never experienced an illness. Doctors, relatives, friends and 'miracle fuzzies' generously share all they know. But not one of them knows what it feels like to actually have the illness. None of them know your fears, your pain, or how it feels to be at the mercy of a disease and helpless in the face of an overwhelming situation.

They all make big talk while you get smaller and smaller. I hated it when someone gave me their piece of advice on how to fight back the illness. And when I was given instructions on how to train my muscles in order not to lose muscle mass too quickly, I thought to myself, "Please shut up right now!" Although I was inwardly boiling I would calmly say, "I don't have a problem with my muscles, I have a problem with my nervous system!" It occurred to me over and over again that people had no idea about my feelings, my pain, and my torment.

But I also knew that they meant no harm. Even the specialists who told me that I suffered from MS had no idea. NOT ONE of them had MS and was able to feel into my body. For every one of the so- called experts it was impossible to imagine how it is to have no feeling in your right arm. My arm was there but it was cold, stiff and numb. It was the same as having no arm at all. Only someone else with the same illness is likely to understand you. All the others just talk about it. Don't let just anyone convince you of something.

Decide independently for yourself, listen to yourself. Even if there is silence at first, you will gradually develop a sense for listening to your body, and to your inner voice. We have simply 'unlearnt' to listen!

Increasing reduction

In 2009 I went for treatment to a centre specialising in neurological conditions. At that stage I was very **sensitive to pressure** and even the softest mattress at this centre was too hard for me. I had to have my own special mattress brought from home so that I could sleep there. After four weeks I realised that the therapy was far too exhausting for me and that I hadn't benefitted much. The therapists had all been friendly and cooperative but the whole program was just too much for me.

I was glad to be home again. After that experience I never went for another treatment of that kind again. While at the neurology centre I was thoroughly examined and one doctor detected a malposition of my pelvis and right leg (especially the knee). Because of the slow degeneration of muscles in my right leg my **gait** had deteriorated and in order to compensate I was increasingly pushing with my knee. The consequence was an arthrosis in my right knee which accelerated rapidly. I therefore had to wear a **leg splint** over my whole leg to relieve the knee. *See picture 2 in photo gallery.*

After the treatment at the neurological centre I was issued with a medical certificate for my condition. I simply couldn't go any further.

I still made a few attempts to go to work but I was incapable of working, and so I had to finally retire.

2010 was a quite a year. I had to overcome various personal crisis; a separation, my retirement and the move into a new building with facilities for handicapped persons. Special facilities had to be installed in the flat such as a bed where I could lie down and get up independently, and holding ropes hanging from the ceiling etc.

The retirement put me on a **psychological** slide on a one-way down; in the end only the Grim Reaper waits. I felt like I had failed, was worthless and useless. Then something else occurred to me: I was utterly vulnerable, attackable. This came as a real shock to me.

My separation was another disaster. I somehow had to experience being abandoned because of my illness. Many ill people can't be saved from this sad experience. I can only say, "Where one door closes, another door opens." Such an experience is very painful. But don't give up because of it. There are people out there who are not frightened off by illness.

Bouts of depression were very common during this time. The illness cost me my job, my family, my flat, all my money, and a lot more still to come.

In 2010 I needed a **wheelchair** for distances of more than 50 m. At first I had a chair that needed to be pushed, but then in my over eagerness I bought an electrical wheelchair for more independence. It turned out to be a piece of rubbish and completely useless as due to the loss of the use of my right arm I wasn't able to drive it on my own anyway. Later I got a good classical electronic wheelchair from the health insurance. *See picture 5 in photo gallery.*

In 2011 I met my current life partner, Petra. She knew about my clearly visible physical illness, and yet she chose me.

A glimmer of hope, then disappointment

At this point I decided to visit the general hospital in Vienna again to ask if there were any new findings on MS. I was really driven by a fear of ending up in a wheelchair forever. But the doctors made it clear once again that there was no known cure for MS, and that as my disease progressed, there was no medication that would change the situation.)

For MS patients suffering with flare ups or relapses there were various drugs on offer, but for me there was nothing! Could it be any worse? I thought I had already reached the bottom only to find a deeper hole to fall into.

But the doctors gave me a small glimmer of hope by offering me the chance to participate in a clinical study for a new remedy. In other words, I was to be a guinea pig.

"Okay," I thought to myself, "you are already standing with your back to the wall, how could things get worse?" So I agreed and was given an untested drug named *Fampyra*. It was supposed to improve my walking and help my vertigo.

I started my term as guinea pig in the study. Within two weeks my walking had improved and my vertigo wasn't as bad anymore. Hope and euphoria took hold and I thought that from now on the trend would only be upwards. Sure I wasn't able to walk the distances I had managed before, but I was able to walk more independently.

Every other week I went to the general hospital and reported on whatever small or significant progress I had made and got a further supply of 'miracle pills'. A few months later, while at the hospital I got the bad news that the study had been cancelled without replacement. I was given sufficient pills for a further two weeks and after that it was over for me.

My world started to collapse. What should I do now? I didn't have medication anymore! I asked myself why research on this medication, which had really helped me, had suddenly been cancelled. It had also helped others participating in the study. So why then this abrupt cancellation? They told me, "The medication is simply too expensive!" I couldn't understand it. How could an effective remedy suddenly be too expensive for a human life? For someone suffering with MS?

I got the answer a few months later: The pharmaceutical industry wouldn't make enough profit with it from us, the MS-patients! Sounds hard? Well it is. And it's the truth!

The health insurance industry was not willing to carry the cost of a long-term medication, and for a private person the medication would not be affordable. Of course it has to be worth it, and everyone has his financial constraints. But clearly, so do the health insurance companies. I had no more money (having spent it all on 'miracle healers') so my limit had already been reached. All sorts of accusations arose in me. How can the health insurance industry not want to bear the cost of medication that heals an illness?

The sad and shocking truth is that it's all about the money. The pharmaceutical industry does nothing for free even if they appear to care about the wellbeing of people. I did not think about such things as I had always been a healthy person, and even when I did get ill I got a prescription from the doctor and everything was OK. But being critically affected, and experiencing so directly that my own life is too expensive, one starts to see things differently; a realization dawned, a rethinking and an awakening began.

Down again

That was when I started to educate myself by studying my disease and learning about the general mechanics and the nature of the body.

I read everything I could lay my hands on and compared it over and over again with scientific studies. I wanted to understand my own body. I had nothing else to do so I studied excessively. It became a kind of pastime. I didn't think about a cure or a later destiny where I would share my knowledge with others. Studying helped against the pain and the extreme boredom.

By July 2012 I was bedridden and lying an average of 23 hours a day. Problems in my back and legs made sitting too painful. Due to lack of movement my right arm and leg had become very swollen and the accumulation of lymphatic fluid caused excruciating pain. To make things a bit more bearable I wore compression stockings on my right arm and on both legs.

All in all I quite literally lay in bed for around 1½ years, and almost exclusively on my left side. Lying on my right caused unbearable pain. Lying on my back was possible but only for short periods of time.

During this period I **gained a lot of weight** *(see picture 3 in the photo gallery).* I simply ate and didn't move at all. I ate much more than I needed purely out of frustration. I am 180 cm tall and my body weight increased from 80 kg to 90 kg and then from 100 kg to 110 kg, until I didn't step onto my scale anymore. The only kind of 'walking' I did was going to the toilet, and doing the most basic, necessary things to exist.

For one and a half years this was my view of the world. Did I ever mention the **ceiling crane**? I needed a ceiling crane to help me get out of bed. In the beginning the rope was just a support tool but it very soon became a must-have in order to move any part of my body, and to get up from bed. *(See picture 4A and picture 4B in the photo gallery).*

Shower and washing myself was a major feat of strength. Without help it wouldn't have been possible at all. Almost nothing was possible without help!

Just one way out

The doctors had given up on me, and at this point, with absolutely no prospects at all, I wished for a quick death from a heart attack or a stroke. Excessive and unhealthy eating was in some way part of my plan to end my life. 'Life' was not the name I would give the situation I was in. It was a slow wasting away, a gradual degeneration to be followed by a slow, painful death. It did not mean that I had given up; I simply didn't have an alternative.

But something in me always had hope. Some small voice in me said, "Stay strong! This is not the end. You still have a task ahead of you!" I didn't understand it as 'hope' at the time. I didn't understand the point of the whole thing at all. I had been robbed of absolutely everything, I was left with nothing.

What could I still have tried with a body so lame and sick, and completely dependent on help? I could basically do nothing other than move my right leg and my left arm. It was Christmas time and I asked myself "What does it mean? What hope? What beginning?" Those thoughts were little seeds, like the sprouts of a plant.

Over all the following days I was beset with anguishing, confusing thoughts, and there was nothing I could do to avoid them. They kept returning again and again. I was torn between giving up and surviving.

Suddenly, on New Year's Eve, a flash of inspiration struck me. It was absolutely crazy. A totally absurd thought: Not everything was completely hopeless. I AM able to DO something… I can try to get **HEALTHY** again!

Thinking inwardly I said to myself, "If I am not able to die, then there has to be a way back to health! What is stopping me from trying to get healthy again? What else do I have to do?" I first had to completely re-organise and reconstruct my whole life in my head, in order to find a new meaning for life. Of course I was afraid of failing, but

The real failure lies in not even trying!

To wait for a miracle, in my opinion, was a waste of time. Why should I be able to achieve something that even the doctors have no solution for? I don't know. There is nothing special about me. I am just like everyone else.

The only thing I have is an unbendable will. If I decide on something I will follow my goal to the end. MS is said to be incurable but I, the ordinary chap from next door, am facing the problem. Why? Because there is NOTHING else to do for me!

I am neither religious nor particularly esoteric. Sure there are certain concepts I don't understand and some do seem to be a bit more than just mumbo jumbo. For instance, I consider the simple little daisy to be a scientific mystery. There, in the meadow with soil that lacks calcium, daisies are able to grow. Typically, plants get their nutrients and minerals from the soil through their roots. The mystery is that daisies have a lot of calcium in them. And no one knows for sure where they get their calcium. The soil doesn't offer this element. And there are many more such little mysteries, but let's continue with my wondrous change of heart.

The foundation was laid. The decision had been made. All I had to do now was to find the right path. Yes, you understood it, the right road: I wanted…., no, I *had* to get healthy again. I just didn't know how. Interestingly, the decision alone was essential. Just when you start looking for something you will most certainly find a way. In the state of hopelessness many people never even start the search, so the many hidden possibilities are never revealed to them. Just a few months later my path led me to Helmuth Matzner, to whom I will refer in a later chapter.

In the **bonus resources** page at the end of the book you will find links, some of which can be downloaded. There are also on-site videos about my ordeal and my road to success.

CHAPTER 3: THE START OF MY THIRD LIFE

Or
What does one need in order to become healthy?

The year 2014

My third started at the beginning of 2014. In this chapter I will describe some of the decisions and choices which helped me onto the road to recovery, especially during these early days of change. Sure, I am not completely healed and back to my normal health, but I have certainly regained some control over my life, and a large degree of independence. My health improved significantly during this phase, I started to 'live' again, and for this I am truly grateful.

My friend the diary

Following my 'change of heart' and the decision to regain my health, I continued to do as I had done before, lying in bed. Other than watching TV, reading or studying something I didn't have much else to do. Eventually I gave some thought to my current state and wondered what I could actually do to improve my health.

I wrote my New Year's Resolution in my diary:

"Today is the beginning of my third life!"

I can sincerely recommend to everyone to keep a diary. Not only to refer back to what happened a year ago, but to remain active and alert. It is not necessary to write every day. Although it is actually the regularity of putting something down on paper that is in itself very helpful.

As long as I am able to write I know I am alive and able to think. I had always been afraid of stagnating altogether.

Why do handcraft despite the handicaps?

Besides writing a diary I started doing handcraft as well as I was able to with my limited fine motor skills and hand co-ordination. I had always been a craftsman and very proud of being able to everything on my own. From having two partially- skilled hands I now only had one. But this didn't scare me away from doing handcrafts. My right hand was replaced by certain ingenious tools which I had built for myself. As a trained toolmaker I was able to build 'substitute fingers' for myself. That may sound funny but it was necessary. I constructed pliers and clamps which I could hold and operate with my left leg.

Petra had to help me initially as I wasn't able to do certain sawing and drilling work alone. But as soon I was ready with my 'tool making' I wanted to manage everything on my own. This was very important for me and my psyche. I started creating rings out of paper which I had seen in a video on the internet. An artist called Jeremy May invented paper jewellery and I thought "I want to do this too!"

I didn't want to earn money from it, rather to take up a challenge. The video didn't show how the rings were made, only how beautiful they looked in the end. Through learning by doing and with a lot of persistence I was finally able to produce my first self-made paper ring. This hobby was affordable, cheap, and a physical and intellectual challenge for me. I needed a lot of time for one ring but it was fun doing it over and over again.

The whole time I worked with just one hand, my left hand – filing, drilling, polishing and coating. Just one ring engaged me fully for about 25 hours.

After sitting and filing for two hours at a stretch my whole body hurt, but I was still glad that I could achieve something, although after such strenuous work I had to lie down for the rest of the day and recover.

I had nothing else to do. Yet I was able to do a lot while lying down. One can hardly believe what is all possible when lying down. It is even possible to file, grind and polish while lying down, and all this with only one hand. (*See picture 6 in photo gallery*)

I needed a challenge or a task otherwise I wouldn't have been able to endure the seemingly endless stretches of time for much longer. When one gets sick and tired of watching TV, reading, lying down, looking out the window and counting the hours, one is happy to experience whatever pain or discomfort from doing crafts. It was far more fulfilling than just waiting for some doctor to produce 'miracle pills'. By this stage I had been through enough, I didn't want to grapple with everything on an intellectual level. I just wanted to be busy, with my body, doing something satisfying and constructive.

My hunger for knowledge
I made one mistake. During this time I had learnt a lot about the body, about people, the processes of life and health, but I hadn't yet applied it to myself. Up to now I had successfully managed to avoid the issue by writing everything off to 'destiny', where I simply had to wait patiently for whatever life imposed on me, and accept that there was no suitable medicine on the market.

I read several medical journals and watched DVDs about getting healthy. There is a very good book by Bruce Lipton, PhD. ***The biology of belief: Unleashing the Power of Consciousness, Matter & Miracles / The Wisdom of your Cells: How your beliefs control your body.*** This book is about our body's cells being able to repair all ailments. In addition to this book there is also a DVD which explains visually in a simple way what the human body, more specifically our body's cells, are able to achieve.

The key message of this book is that we are all regulated by our environment. Our cells, and us as whole human beings, exist in accordance with the laws of nature. Changing our environment will mean a change in life. It was very exciting coming to realise that our environment is largely responsible for how we feel.

The body's cells can be healed if one is willing to start caring for them. If we pay attention to the environment of our cells we should be able to intervene proactively and effect significant changes. Of course this would not be possible overnight, but then most of us are looking for something that works instantly. Ultimately, quick fixes don't exist, it's all nonsense, but the pharmaceutical industry continues to promote them. It is similar to TV spots where a dirty stove is shown, which then sparkles after only one wipe with the 'miracle cleaning agent'. Who really takes it seriously?

Where does the fight for health start?
Whoever has acted against his body causing illness to creep in over the decades has to accept that it will need time to heal. Each body has its own weak areas where disease is most likely to occur. Mine was MS.

Whoever made the excuse, "I know someone who smoked for over 50 year and didn't get ill!" is mistaken. If you look closely you will see hospitals full of these 'supposedly healthy' people. The truth is blurred because we don't visit hospitals all the time. We ignore the truth to avoid seeing it. Everyone has his weak point which we deny until the disease reminds us how vulnerable we are. I don't mean to be an alarmist, please see this rather as a wake-up call to do something NOW before it is too late.

From this point on I wanted to get healthy again! But how? I had no plan and no idea what to implement, how to achieve it practically. To my mind I had lived a healthy life prior to becoming ill. I neither smoked nor drank alcohol. Sure, as a young man I had smoked a little but I quit a long time before getting ill. Stress is another factor which must be taken seriously. Additional triggers to my getting ill were most certainly consuming fast-foods, energy-dinks and Cola.

What I ate and drank wasn't always the healthiest choice. At that stage I wasn't aware of the consequences. Besides, becoming sick was simply a 'destiny' thing; something that one was not in control of oneself.

I checked my attitudes to life and my life-style and began to notice certain thought patterns which were clearly not conducive to good health.

I always fought against the disease, but against who or what was I actually fighting? MS is an autoimmune disease. It is a disease where your own body turns against itself. If my immune system turns against me and my answer is to 'fight' back, then a war would start and I would certainly be the loser.

If your body is trying to tell you something and your response is to fight it, what's the point of that?

The best way to demonstrate this is to stand in front of the mirror and slap yourself. Let's see who has the necessary persistence to win the fight. Have fun figuring out who will be stronger.

Our thoughts are the key – but only the right ones!

Pressure generates counter-pressure!
Fighting against yourself doesn't help!

Instead of fighting we should ask our body, "Why? Why are you acting against me? What can I do for you? How can I possibly help you to get healthy?" No healthy body wants to die. Only our own abuse of it can lead it there. We are the ones generating a resistance to our body's needs and acting against its life force. We are the ones damaging our bodies by smoking and drinking cola and alcohol, taking drugs, eating the wrong foods and poisoning ourselves with harmful thoughts. We even abuse our bodies with extreme sport, too little sleep, insufficient inner peace, harmful hygiene (eg. antiperspirants with aluminium), etc. I only mention things which we ourselves are able to take responsibility for. There are several other body pollutants but I won't say anything about these particular culprits at this stage.

During this time, looking at my life more inwardly, many astonishing insights arose. I questioned all my beliefs and worked through everything I thought was important. I was honest with myself and I removed the rose coloured glasses. There was much inner upheaval.

I went through a total re-evaluation of my attitudes and priorities, and a complete reorganising of my thinking.

Sadly, I had to accept that I had deceived myself for a long time. But there was now an end in sight and I began to live with the attitude, "Sure, I have certainly done some stupid things in the past but from now on I could try to do them better!" MS didn't hit me out of the blue - it was the consequence of my unhealthy lifestyle. I would recommend everyone reflect on themselves and get to know yourself better.

The first new thing to appear is a thought. If this thought is worth continuing with, then an idea may arise out of it. If this idea still feels good, then deeds can follow. But consider the following: You have to take the responsibility for the whole process.

I had never noticed it previously, but during those long periods just lying in bed I observed something: I recognised that my body was on the same level as my head. Why would that be important? When one stands upright then the head is the highest point. We therefore look down on our body from above. And this is exactly the way we treat it most of the time - from up above. The head gives a command and the body has to follow like a good slave regardless of the consequences. But shouldn't we actually be living in harmony with it? Giving it equal regard and consideration?

Your body doesn't speak the same language as you do. It has no voice and can only communicate with you through its feelings. If we don't develop the sense to 'hear' it then a disease will follow.

And if hearing its call doesn't force you to rethink your situation then the last option for your body is to die.

We CAN learn to listen to the body and start sensing what it needs, and how to treat it in a respectful and considerate way. Only then will we be able to avoid or cure diseases. After all, our body is the only 'home' in which we live on earth. So we should treat it with more respect.

If we are honest with ourselves we will have to admit that it's not the body that is harming us, it is our behaviour that is harming the body to the point of becoming ill. We are responsible for becoming ill. If the body is no longer able to function in a proper way we try to force it, we start to fight against it. We should think very seriously about this attitude!

CHAPTER 4: MY PHYSICAL CONDITION IN JANUARY 2014

In this chapter I describe my physical condition as it was at the beginning of 2014, being the start of my 'third life'. I made some videos of my home and general environment to give you an idea of how I lived at the time. You can retrieve these videos through a link in the **bonus resources** page.

January 2014: My **right hand** and fingers are cold, stiff and too swollen to do anything with at all. I have learnt to do everything with my left hand. I see this as a great advantage because after using my right hand for most things (being a right handed person), it meant that once I gained the use of my right hand again I would be able to use both hands equally well. I have learnt to recognise benefits in everything.

The **right arm** itself is pretty useless (max. 10% useage); my biceps, triceps and shoulder muscles are all weak so it is difficult to lift anything. I can't raise my right arm over my head. In addition, the muscles in my shoulder have shortened in such a way that even physiotherapy can't rehabilitate it. I also have **lime** deposits in my right shoulder which make larger movements very painful. The skin is mostly feels numb and in certain areas it is also extremely sensitive. Altogether: a total waste of an arm.

My **left leg** is partially paralyzed. With the exception of the thigh muscle the leg is lame. The foot hangs limp and the calf muscles, Achilles heel and shinbone muscles are paralyzed. Everything is numb from my toes to my knee.

Due to the lack of muscle my knee has shifted out of position. Furthermore, there is a strong arthrosis in my right knee. I have to wear a **leg splint** in order to walk even a few steps. It helps in lifting the foot and stabilizing the leg.

The front **thigh muscle** has about 50% functionality but the back thigh muscle is slack, so I have a lot of pain in the leg whether I lie down or walk. Stepping on the left foot is particularly painful. The whole foot feels like I am standing on a bed of nails.

The **right hip** has only 10% of its function. Lifting the right leg is impossible. Through standing for long periods the hips have shifted. When I feel good I am able to walk about 10 m with the help of the splint and a walking stick. But I need many stops in between. For everything else I need a wheelchair.

On bad days I am not able to walk at all as due to the vertigo I am constantly giddy and prone to falling. So I avoid walking wherever possible. If I fell and injured myself when no one was around I would be totally helpless. So I only walk when it is absolutely necessary. I have two alternatives for leaving my flat: either I go by car (Petra drives) or I take the wheelchair.

I avoid most things simply because it is too dangerous. When I go out by car I won't walk about anywhere. My radius is 5 m and any more than that then Petra has to push me in my wheelchair. I hate this alternative! If I fell I would need help because without help I wouldn't be able to stand up again. For this reason I installed an electrical rope hoist between my living room and my bed room.

If I were to fall when I was in the flat I would use it to get back up on my feet again. I am not even able to close my eyes whilst standing as I would lose my balance immediately.

My abdominal muscles are very weak, as are the muscles on the right side of my back. I hold my body upright as well as I can with the left side of my torso. Tension and pain from **postural defects** have become normal for me.

Except for a few skin irritations **the left** leg is unharmed. For this reason I am still able to 'walk', or whatever one might call it. The left arm and the left shoulder are completely dysfunctional. I could act in a zombie movie in Hollywood, I would fit in perfectly well with all the weirdos. They also drag themselves around or schlepp themselves across the floor. Yes, I look like a zombie when I walk. Maybe I should apply for a role in Hollywood. Me, a movie star…?!

Unfortunately I have a **weak pelvic floor** which means that I literally drive from toilet to toilet.

Riding my exercise bike is impossible because of **coordination disorder** in my legs. Standing on just one leg, whether it is the right leg or the left one, is impossible.

The **regeneration time** after taking a shower or doing some other exhausting activity is at least four hours. I am quite wrecked after any physical exertion and need to sleep for an hour or two to regenerate. That means I have to lie down after every physical activity to recharge my batteries.

I don't recover whilst sitting. Sitting is only possible for short periods as after an hour or so it becomes very painful and I have to lie down anyway. If I don't lie down and rest my whole body then it hurts the next day. Although lying down is very painful too.

I **get very tired** after only a few minutes of effort, which soon turns into exhaustion. This exhaustion is overwhelming when it happens. If I didn't have something to sit or lie on immediately then I would collapse on the spot.

My **body's energy** level is generally very low. Walking, standing, getting dressed, showering and going to the toilet are all extremely strenuous for me. It wears me down to exhaustion and I have to lie down to recover.

The high **temperatures** in summer are very difficult. I don't leave my flat because I cannot bear the heat and sunshine. MS conditions cannot tolerate heat.

During the first years I had no problem with my **eyes**. Problems occurred gradually over time in the form of dry eyes. Sometimes things close to me appear very blurred. Reading is only possible at a distance of about 40 – 50 cm. I use a magnifying glass to read the newspaper and to read text on the screen of my laptop I have to enlarge the letters.

I am also very sensitive to **pressure** and need a special mattress or else I wouldn't be able to sleep. I can't stay overnight in a strange bed such as in a hotel.

My right arm and right leg are always swollen due to lack of movement.

The accumulation of lymph fluid is very painful. I have to wear **compression stockings** on the right arm and both legs.

Because of lying for long periods of time and eating too much my **weight** has increased to 110 kg.

Taking a shower has become a mammoth challenge that I couldn't manage without help.

I have **cramps** and **spasms** with almost every movement. Especially when getting out of bed. In the morning, with only the slightest movement, I get extreme cramps and continuous spasms in my whole body. When getting up from a chair I get spasms right away, and then the cramps come.

For 30 years I have had recurring **eczema** on different parts of my body. Currently I have an annoying eczema behind both ears.

30 years ago I also contracted **psoriasis** on my whole body including my face and head. It was often so bad that it bled and I had scabs all over my body. Sometimes, after the administration of Cortisone, the psoriasis would disappear for a period of time. Most affected were my elbows, knees, the hairline of my forehead, between the eyebrows, my nostrils, my upper lip and the sides of my cheeks. (*See picture 7 in photo gallery*)

For many years I suffered from **renal colic** which is extremely painful and would last several days at a time. A total of six kidney stones were passed. They were the size of pebbles and caused enormous pain while passing.

Anyone who has had such an experience will be able to identify with the pain I am referring to.

For years I have been taking a medicine called Lioresal. I take a daily dose of 125 mg. Lioresal is a muscle relaxant and helps to prevent or lessen spasms and cramps. The recommended daily dose is only 25 mg. I take more than the recommended dose but without this drug I wouldn't be able to sleep due to constant cramps and spasms.

I have reached my absolute pain threshold and I can't imagine crossing it. Strong painkillers are part of everyday life for me. 48 mg of Hydal is my daily dose. For you information, 48 mg of Hydal is the normal dose for cancer patients in their final stage.

Like many MS-sick people I have **fatigue-syndrome**. This means chronic exhaustion which is not caused by physical effort. One feels faint, weak and completely exhausted without doing anything at all.

The above is a summary of my condition as in January 2014. Now I want to make big changes in my life. I made the resolve on New Year's Eve. The next thing was to find the road that would lead me there. One that is right for me, the one that will work for the person I am. It has to be a road that suits me. Regardless of the roads that other people take. I can only break new ground for myself and go in a new direction with my own steps, one at a time.

CHAPTER 5: THE NECESSARY MOTIVATION AND GOALS

Give yourself a chance

Try it! Lift your body, your soul, your spirit, and GIVE YOURSELF A CHANCE! No one other than yourself can do it for you. The first thing I did was to formulate a basic strategy for myself, consisting of several steps. One of these steps was based on the motto: Motivate yourself every day!

Dear reader, it is without doubt the most vital tool: to motivate yourself every day!

It is the single most important attitude for a real breakthrough, and essential for success and survival! If one is not able to motivate oneself every day then one has absolutely no chance! The one who gives up on himself crashes! Nobody is able to motivate you like you can motivate yourself. If others (friends, family etc.) try it will not have the same effect, and you will soon experience their motivation as an irritating, distracting and annoying pressure. And as a result you will probably close yourself off inwardly.

For this reason you need to motivate yourself directly, no matter how! Figure out your own strategies. Everything is allowed. After all, it's your life that's at stake! I had weak periods just like everyone else, but I had a clear and strong dream which helped me to lift myself up again each time.

First: focus on success by setting realistic daily goals.

It is best if you approach it in a relaxed way. How do you relax? Perhaps music, Yoga or exercising may work for you – they worked well for me. Tai-Chi can bring peace to body and mind as can any kind of meditation. If you are relaxed and able to look into yourself, the right thoughts and feelings will find their way to you. Once you achieve a sense of serenity you can start to formulate your dreams and goals.

It would be important to set goals in such a way that you are able to reach them. In the beginning I set mini targets for myself, consciously. I wanted to train myself for success. This 'becoming and staying successful' was very important. If I continuously failed my goals because I set them too high, then I could lose my motivation, and failure would become pre-programmed, I would anticipate failure.

But if I set my goals in a realistic way so that they are reachable in the beginning, then my mind-set is one of expectancy and achievement, and one becomes accustomed to this. One has to habituate oneself to success very slowly and carefully, because with a disease like MS one has constantly to cope with defeats. But if one programs oneself for achievement, then the odd defeat isn't that bad.

I increased my daily targets slowly over time, as needed by my mind and body. In the beginning I set the goals very low to be sure to reach them so that I would experience successes on a daily basis.
It is precisely the small steps which take one forward; step by step, week by week, month by month. Never give up.

Your mind-set will change to winning mode, but only with time.

Bigger goals

Once you are coping with the small goals you can start setting the bigger goals. They should also be realistic and reachable. When we are in winning mode then nothing can stop us. What is the sense of setting a goal that you cannot reach? It only brings frustration and dejection. If this happens too often I get despondent. But I didn't want to lie flat and helpless - I know that 'place' only too well. I wanted to be a part of life again and to regain my joy. All the more reason to not set myself on a path to failure.

However, there are some important goals which are unreachable. But you don't have to put all your hopes on them immediately. In the beginning, small successes are essential for motivation. If my mind is already adjusted to winning and achievement then I will deal with failures in a different way. Once the daily goals have been achieved one can move onto weekly goals and then monthly targets. I wouldn't go further because one has to remain flexible in case something elementary changes. And that may happen quite often. It also depends on one's living conditions. Some goals may even need an annual plan. In my case it was not necessary to plan for a whole year.

If you reach your goals day by day over a longer time span, your motivation is strengthened. 'Lectures' from those around you are not so annoying anymore. I always avoided cynics, critics and grumblers, and especially the 'know-it-alls'.

I am sure you know what I mean! I was often told not to be too disappointed if something didn't work out.

Such statements rather dragged me down and then I didn't feel like making any effort because in my mind I was now expecting to failure. The only thing that helped was to stay away from negative people for as long as possible.

Only when I got very much stronger was I immune to their 'advice', and then they couldn't harm me anymore. No one meant it in a bad way, no one wanted to harm me, but they simply didn't recognise how much they eroded my courage and determination. Even when I did improve, their well-meant advice wouldn't stop. Some people just are like that. We only have to learn how to deal with them. Such people don't understand what you have already achieved and that it isn't possible to be disappointed anymore.

If you remain focussed and diligent you will reach your goals every day! This will in turn motivate you more and you will gain strength from your successes. This 'reprogramming' is slow but there are great rewards. The fruits which you will harvest on an emotional level will be that much sweeter with increased physically health and wellness.

A saying which I found helpful:
"Success is measured by our defeats and how we deal with them."

I have had enough of defeats. Now I want success.

My '5-S' Strategy for self-motivation
How does one achieve constant motivation? It is as easy as it is difficult. It is easy if one has a clear dream and the right goals. But it is difficult to set the right goals.

I noticed that I could only become motivated once I had reflected, revised and clarified my mental attitude towards myself. I therefore created what I call the '5-S' strategy:

'5-S' refers to:
- **Self-confidence**
- **Self-awareness**
- **Self-esteem**
- **Self-love**
- **Self-worth**

I considered the 5-S strategy over and over again and came to the realisation that I had previously had a completely incorrect picture of myself. In order to help myself I had to start with a healthy and positive attitude towards myself.

It is this simple: If I don't like myself because my body is too large or because it shows some other 'deficiency', then why would I want to help it? Subconsciously we reject ourselves, we disrespect and reject our bodies and then nothing can change, nothing new can come.

For example: I look at myself in the mirror and ask myself, "Do I like this person in the mirror?" If the answer is "No!", then your subconscious mind says, "So why shall I help this body now?" It is exactly this attitude that perpetuates the situation. That is why it's extremely important to reflect on the 5-S as honestly as possible before starting anything. I am not able to change anything about my body if my basic attitude towards myself is negative!

Creating the right dream

If, like me, you are standing with your back to the wall, there is only one direction: forwards. Even though it may not be that easy.

After I revised my own 5-S I spent hours and days searching for a dream worth pursuing. I had many dreams all of which I dismissed over and over again, because they were not strong enough to defy and overcome all the obstacles lying on the path ahead of me.

Finally I found it! My own 'wonderful dream' which would help me to gain the strength and focus I would need. I had to give it all of me, all my effort and focus, every single day. From then on I looked neither left nor right. I didn't allow myself to be distracted and worked steadily day after day on myself. I forgot everything around me and I saw instead every single little change that occurred in me.

I wrote everything down; every small progress, every step backwards, simply everything. I was used to writing because I had kept a diary (see excerpts in later chapters), but this kind of writing was new. Every day I sank into deep contemplation and started listening very closely to what my body was telling me. With time I regained a positive and alert sense for my body and my condition, which I had lost during the long illness.

Another very important discovery was that knowledge and understanding are two different things. If I 'know' something it doesn't necessarily mean I understand it. This was a real life-changing discovery for me. A simple example is where everyone 'knows' that smoking is bad for the health, and yet many people continue to smoke.

If people truly understood why it was unhealthy, then all smokers would immediately quit and there wouldn't be any smokers in the world. Knowledge alone isn't very helpful; you need to really grasp it and understand why!

As a bonus for readers there is a link to a website on the **bonus resources** pages where you can download my daily routine and a work sheet on how to find the 'right dream' and set the 'right goals'. I hope it will help you, as it helped me, and I am looking forward to receiving your feedback.

Second: I had to lose weight

The second thing I had to do was to lose weight. I had to reduce weight to the point where I could carry my own body. But how? I had been lying down, hardly moving, for so long. To even think about doing sports would have been ridiculous. Other than falling, which I did quite regularly, I couldn't claim to have done anything sporty. Rather cheekily I would tell Petra and my friends to please rate my body shape and my facial expressions and tell me their scores!

Since sport wasn't an option I would have to cut down on food. But while that may reduce fat, it brings the danger of losing muscle mass, which was highly risky for me with MS. But it was a risk I had to take. So I started eating less. The result was that I lost some weight and gained some strength. At last I was able to visit the toilet.

What else was there to do! I started studying up on how to lose weight without losing body strength. The internet and diet books offer many explanations, but not everything. I looked for information on how someone like me would be able to lose weight safely.

There is no description in any book on how to lose weight when you are seriously ill. So I dared to start experimenting with 'losing weight in the right way' using the little knowledge I had gained from the internet and books, together with my own intuition. Giving myself time, through experimentation with and observation of my own body, I was able to reduce my weight without losing strength.

Third: Learning to move properly

The third thing I had to learn was how to move properly again. Due to lying flat for so long my body had become stiff. I had unlearnt how to do simple things such as walk, bend over, stretch limbs etc. I had to almost start from zero again. Without the right motivation this wouldn't have been possible.

Because I had done Yoga and Tai-Chi previously I thought this would be a good way to start. I tried as best I could to do some of the exercises as I remembered them, but it is no exaggeration when I admit that it was the purest horror in the beginning! I had such severe cramps and spasms I was convinced something was going to tear off my body. Sometimes the pain was so bad that I would cry out loud. In such moments the only thing which made me continue was my dream.

I had to stretch and lengthen my arms and legs. Over time the muscles, tendons, everything had shortened and had to be exercised to become flexible and movable again. All movement was painful. The most unpleasant exercise was twisting and stretching my torso. Sadly couldn't continue with the Yoga exercises due to the pain.

The worst thing for me was the fight against tiredness and exhaustion. The long phases of sleep that I needed after every exercise to recover held up me for hours. I could only manage two or three exercises before getting too tired and needing to sleep. I would get tired, pause for two minutes, and then force myself to lift my leg just 5 cm again. Next break. Once again, just once again, until I had done it right. Sometimes I would feel queasy and would have to throw up due to exertion.

Each movement was a fight; not 'against' my body but 'for' my body. I had to regain a degree of fitness in order to be able to walk at least 50 – 100 m. It took months to finally get there, but I knew that I would achieve it someday. Overcoming the pain and exhaustion at the beginning was certainly the hardest thing I have ever had to do in my entire life. I can fully recommend you never give up. The reward is a new life!

At this point I want to thank my darling Petra again. In reality it's not possible to give adequate thanks for the dedication and support given by someone in this way. She helped me through my worst times and stood by my side 24/7. She certainly didn't have an easy life with me, but she never abandoned me.

How to get healthy again?
We now move to the next question, "What can I do in order to become strong and healthy again?" Take a look back over your life's journey to see what had made you sick in the first place. But beware, this means we have to deal with ourselves honestly and grapple with the real truths. This can be a painful process. Sometimes even, extremely painful.

I took a close look at all my 'sins'. I spent a lot of time going back in time and writing down my thoughts and what I remembered. Each detail might be important. One should therefore be prepared to give a lot of time to this process. With such knowledge one can look for specific solutions. I went over every memory of the past 25 years; which foods I had, how much stress I had, the diseases, visits to the dentist, general practitioners, even how often I got cramps in my calves. Everything became important, like collecting and putting together all the pieces of a puzzle.

During this phase of looking back into the past I started with my physical training. I was 'hungry for life' again and so I used everything I could find as a training object. Every movement became an exercise e.g. opening the water bottle, lifting it, and guiding it to my mouth. Even my walk to the toilet was done in a conscious way so that it turned into a training exercise. I wasn't able to hold a spoon with my right hand so the spoon turned into a training object too. I started from ground zero and went the hard way. Because I had found the right dream.

Motivation is everything, and if you want to repair a damaged body you need time. It's not going to happen in a few days. It took me years to get to the point where I had acquired the necessary knowledge and focus in order to get a grip on my reality. But now I had to put it into practice. A lot is possible with the right attitude and the right information. But I must state here: one has to reckon with the fact that there may be certain damages from the medication or the illness itself, which can't be ignored or reversed. These will naturally differ from person to person depending on the illness and the life's circumstances.

When I became strong enough to make basic steps I learnt how to use the shopping trolley; I would just lean on it and off I'd go with some sort of walking moves.

Because my right hand was cold and stiff I couldn't use a walker at home. A shopping trolley provided the chance to rest on it with my upper body and to use my right hand. As you can imagine, there were quite a few funny situations with the shopping trolley. In the beginning I was only able to pull myself along, but I couldn't control the direction. If I happened to have a 'stubborn' trolley which pulled left or right, I simply had to follow it. Then Petra would have to rescue me from half way down some isle I never wanted to traverse in the first place, and redirect the errant trolley back to the fruit and veg section.

For Petra it was less funny. In the beginning she didn't always have time to go searching for me in the shopping mall and she was quite stressed by it. Sometimes I had to stop in the middle, unable to go any further. I would manage a few minutes and then would have to sit down immediately, even in the middle of the shop. After a short break sitting on the floor, or on some pallets with cans or bottles as company, I would continue until the next break.

Although these shopping sprees were initially very exhausting I gradually built up my muscles and endurance. I also enjoyed the chance to socialise again. With time my stamina increased and eventually I became 'master' of my shopping trolley. Then I was able to direct it on my own.

Some people stared at me. There I was, walking like an old man at my age. But I didn't let it distract me. I often responded with a serious look on my face saying, "I was shot in the back during my last robbery."

Some would disappear very quickly while others laughed and the ice would be broken. I often just said, "I am looking for someone who is willing to exchange his body with mine. Are you interested?"

I believe one shouldn't take life too seriously.
In any case, no one has survived it as yet.

CHAPTER 6: HELPFUL NUTRITION

About good health and bad health, food for life or pleasure

There are many good books on health and nutrition and there is a wealth of information on the internet. The problem is that there is nothing for people in my particular situation.

Our reason for eating has become little more than a case of "it tastes so good." Let's consider this attitude. I needed a long time before I was able to admit to myself that I, and no one else, was responsible for eating the types and quantities of food that I had consumed. What I all crammed into myself just because it tasted so good, and not because it was good for me! What kind of response can I expect from my body when I treat it with a complete lack of respect and loads of unhealthy food? We don't fill our cars with the cheapest fuel at the station, we make sure to use the best. So why not do the same with our bodies?

If the boss of a big company pushes us steadily to give our maximum 18 hours a day while paying a minimum wage with no breaks at all, how long would we last? Right! With bad nutrition we do exactly the same thing with our bodies.

A healthy and balanced diet is of the highest importance. What is healthy food? I decided to separate the concept of 'foods/foodstuffs' and 'nutrition'. 'Foods' simply feed the body to keep it alive with the most basic necessities, whereas 'nutrition', as the word suggests, nourish the body. They include the healthy stuff such as fruit and vegetables high in vitamins and enzymes.

I believe this is a very important distinction. We all know that fast foods fill the stomach to a certain degree, but no not actually nourish us. We need healthy, nutritional foods which haven't lost their 'life force' through some or other process or alteration.

Alkaline or acidic
I make a further distinction between so- called 'base-forming' foods and 'acid-forming' foods.

Base-forming food is the most suitable for our body! These are the green foods like fresh vegetables and fruits. The ratio should be about 70% alkaline to about 30% acidic foods.

Grains, sugar, meat and milk products are strong acid-forming foods and are therefore less healthy for the body.

We all think that fruit and vegetables along with cereals (especially the whole grain type), and milk products are healthy. Well, they are not. If we give it some thought we will see why. Fruit and vegetables are undoubtedly healthy, until you consider the agricultural practices of today? You see the use of pesticides, fungicides and herbicides as far as you look. We consume all these sprays and poisons along with the fruit and vegetable. And this we call healthy?

What helped me
With **grains** one has to reckon with the fact that the body receives too many carbohydrates. Grains also contain gluten, lectins and phytic acid.

For people with MS this is a no go! **Gluten and lectins can cause inflammation in the intestines and they promote MS!** Phytic acid produced by grain plants are not meant to be eaten. Strictly speaking, it is a natural herbal pesticide. Grain appeared on our menus only 10,000 years ago. Our digestive system was not used to it previously.

The exception is **cereal sprouts** which are grains in the germinal form. Germinated cereals provide valuable vitamins and enzymes and should form part of every healthy diet. Sprouts contain a hundredfold more vitamin content than un-sprouted corn e.g. vitamin E + 300%, vitamin C +600% and B-vitamin between + 200% to 1200%. Sprouts are real power packs with a wealth of vital substances. Sadly, grain sprouts also contain gluten!

It is very easy to grow sprouts. Petra and I did it on our own. Unfortunately I had to decline them because of the gluten. One just has to water the grains according to their type for between 4 to 12 hours, and then put them through a sieve to drain the surplus water. They need to be rinsed twice a day, and after two or three days one can eat the sprouts. I always put them in the blender with fruit and mixed it into a tasty drink.

A lot of people suffer from gluten intolerance (coeliac disease). You could test yourself by avoiding all gluten- containing foods (wheat, wheat germ, rye, barley, bulgur, but not rice or maize) for three weeks. You may well discover that your allergies, asthma, eczemas and haemorrhoids have improved.

Milk products are not necessarily good for adults. There are many studies which say that milk is harmful for adults. What is milk?

It is a substance created by mothers specifically for their offspring. Milk contains only those nutrients which are valuable for their particular babies. Milk, with its valuable 'turbo-ingredients', is valuable only for those growing babies. Later it becomes redundant. No grown animal drinks milk unless it has been 'educated' by us to do so, such as with cats, and it is apparently dangerous for wild cats. Milk is something of a boost for life. Milk contains growth hormones, but what should grow in an adult? Cancer?

There is research which proves that drinking milk causes acne and other skin diseases. In Africa and Asia, where cow's milk is hardly consumed, they have the lowest osteoporosis rate. 75% of the world's population suffers from lactose intolerance. This finding itself should be cause for concern.

But I don't want to go too much into detail here because this book goes in another direction. There are sufficient studies on milk to prove it is a danger for adults. Simply put, just imagine driving your car at full speed constantly? Your body can't tolerate 'full speed' in the long run either.

Then there is refined sugar. It is the strongest killer of intestinal flora in existence. Refined sugar (sucrose), and sugar products such as like candy, dextrose, fruit sugar, as well as every kind of brown sugar, weakens our intestinal flora. Sugar is the most harmful food for our intestinal flora. Your intestine is a paradise for sugar which generates aggressive and harmful fungi.

Meat also poses a problem due to all the medication, antibiotics and the stress and trauma of the animals whose wretched lives and poor living conditions are retained in the meat. We wonder why antibiotics and other such remedies hardly help even when we need them. We are becoming immune to antibiotics, and you know where that leads!

So which foods can one eat that are safe and healthy? There are many! The point is to eat the right foods consciously and according to the needs of your body.

I don't want to sound like of those 'nutrition gurus' or 'health advocates', but I have to say: **Forget diets!** Diets only makes one frustrated and aggressive. It is important to think in the longer term, and it's important to have fun with it. **Don't turn yourself into an ascetic!**

I decided on the following solution for myself: **Fruit and vegetables only, and wherever possible, organic**. I am often asked what the difference is. Well, an apple is an apple whether it is organic or not. The difference lies in the trace elements such as the essential oils which are produced in an apple. An organic apple (one that is not treated with artificial fertilisers) needs to produce more antibodies (essential oils) to defend itself against a hungry worm needing a nibble. Just like the apple, our own body needs essential oils to strengthen its antibodies. (I won't even mention at this point the direct damage to the body from the fertilisers themselves). Wherever possible, eat organic. If it not available then one has to be satisfied with what is available at the normal supermarket. One also has to be pragmatic because organic products often cost more, and so affordability is a realistic consideration. Keep it simple, clean and affordable.

70% vegetables, 30% fruit. That's what I aim for, for myself. I don't eat meat, milk products or grain products. I don't consider myself a vegetarian because from time to time I will eat **fish**. I prefer sea fish, if possible from the northern seas. I just live as healthily as possible and try to nourish myself to the best of my knowledge. **I refuse meat** altogether because of the poor quality, and because the living and dying conditions of the animals are unacceptable to me; they are treated way below their dignity. In addition, there are other reasons to refuse meat such as high cholesterol, saturated fatty acids, antibiotics and other medications, which are administered as a matter of course, all of which we in turn take into our own bodies.

It is also very important to use **good salt**. Industrial salt is 'purified and refined' at huge expense. In this process around 80 elements are removed from the original salt. Only sodium chloride (NaCl) remains. This refined salt makes it difficult for our kidneys and for excretion, and on top of this it causes a build-up of crystals on bones and our joints which leads to gout, rheumatism, arthritis and arthrosis. The variety of deposits caused by refined salt can lead to a host of other problems within our body. Also be careful with natural sea salt because 80% of the sea salt on offer in supermarkets is also refined, bleached and supplemented with chemical additives. A good salt is rock salt. It is extracted from salt mines. This salt originated millions of years ago, originally as sea salt. Because we all emerged out of the salt water sea and our cells still know this, our bodies are easily able to process and work with this particular salt.

I wanted to show you that there is hope even within a limited budget.

I wanted to offer guidelines for those of you living with apparently hopeless health challenges. This book begins at the point where the doctors give up on their patients, and so the patients feel lost and hopeless as the future seems to offer no prospects for change. Money is no big issue for me. I never had any, except for what I needed to survive. Someone like me who retires early due to disease has no riches to brag about.

A hot tip for good nutrition: The DVD *'Unsere Rückkehr zur Gesundheit'* ('Our return to health', available only in German) by Helmuth Matzner describes in detail why we should avoid meat, grains and milk. I can highly recommend it (see also chapter 12).

Now that you have made good choices in terms of your foods, how you **prepare and cook** it is equally important. Everything heated to over 107.6°F, or has been frozen, has NO MORE ENZYMES in it! But we absolutely need these enzymes! I therefore suggest we eat our food as raw as possible. If you do, enzymes and vitamins remain unchanged.

Also of importance are **vitamins, minerals, trace elements, amino acids** and **essential oils**. But only those of a **high absorption** and **bioavailability**. There are several minerals and vitamins which cannot be used or processed by the body. Either they need help through an addition substances or supplements in order for the body to be able to use the chemical compound.

An example: The vitamins A, D, E and K are fat-soluble.

If you think you are doing something good for your body by renouncing fat in order to lose weight, you actually do more harm than good. Another example is magnesium: There are several magnesium compounds but only one of them, **magnesium chloride-hexahydrate**, is properly absorbed and effectively utilized by the body. Other compounds need 'help' or they will not be absorbed at all. A hint: I didn't drink the magnesium chloride-hexahydrate, I made footbaths with it. If you drink it you run the risk of getting diarrhoea! In any case the body isn't able to absorb more than 30% of magnesium when taking it internally. In the case of a footbath there is 100% absorption and no danger of diarrhoea. I learnt this from experience, through various experiments. **Never take magnesium together with calcium!** Calcium immediately displaces the magnesium and the body has to excrete it unused. Why the health industry continues to sell this combination of minerals in effervescent powders is a mystery to me. Is it sheer profiteering, or ignorance?

I always imagined it like this: If one wants to build a house one needs things like sand, cement, lime and bricks. Are these substances automatically found at the construction site (analogous to amino acids and minerals in the body)? No, it takes workers to distribute these materials in the right way to the right places. If everything would become mixed up and every worker simply did whatever he wanted to do then the project would be in a state of chaos. Therefore there is a boss on the top who monitors everything and has the plan and assigns everything in the right quantities to the right place, and who monitors for necessary changes. Vitamins and enzymes work in a similar way in our bodies.

Over weeks and months I grappled with the challenge of finding the right organic dietary supplements, with an acceptable composition and ratio of ingredients. I spent a lot of time researching, attending lectures and experimenting with how to use these substances in the best way possible, and safe for my body and particular condition. One can't just do things ad hoc and pour down one's throat anything that may appear healthy, because 'a lot of something good has to be good!'

There is a 'right amount' for everything. And a right combination. Everything has to add up. Someone who takes too much of one thing can actually put himself in danger! There are vitamins, minerals and trace elements which, when overdosed, can cause more damage than be of any use. One should take these dangers seriously.

Salads. I love any kind of salad. With good vinegar and oil. Salad is highly recommended. I also enjoy eating potatoes. Since I changed my diet to healthy-only foods I have never starved. There is an enormous variety of fruit and vegetables on the market.

Instead of boiling I use a **steam cooker** to warm the foods. There are a couple of foods which I don't eat raw. Unfortunately enzymes are lost even with a steam cooker, but the vital substances survive to a large extent. If one boils vegetables in the conventional way many vital substances are leached out. With gentle steam cooking those substances survive. Also a lot of good dishes can also be prepared in a pan. For this I only use coconut oil. Coconut oil tolerates heat best because of its high smoke point from 348.8°F.

I became accustomed to preparing a **fruit smoothie** for myself each morning. Firstly, it subdues the desire to eat sweets and secondly, it provides me with a lot of vitamins, minerals and enzymes. I designed a few mixtures which taste really good.

Another important subject is 'green nutrition' in the form of barley, grass powder, spirulina, chlorella and various other forms of grain grasses because they provide valuable chlorophyll. Why is green nutrition so important for us? We all know that herbs and plants contain a lot of healing substances which is why they are referred to the medicinal plants.

A very good book on this topic is '*The Green Foods Bible – Could Green Plants Hold the Key to Our Survival?*' by David Sandoval.

Besides their healing attributes, green plants and herbs are also base-forming foods. These are essential for our bodies.

Of course one is allowed to eat **acid-forming** foods as well. But only in moderation. Why? If we eat too many acid-forming foods then the body has to counteract the acid. It therefore takes minerals such as calcium, magnesium etc. from our bones and tissues to neutralise the acids. In the long run this leads to a loss of minerals in our bodies which then cause a negative impact on our health. This steady exploitation can lead to chronic disease over time. One can best recognise it by looking at our teeth. Indications in the mouth of acid build up and poor diet are caries, gingivitis and other diseases. Furthermore, an acidic environment in the body supports the growth of aggressive fungi and harmful bacteria.

Unfortunately our pharmaceutical industry would seem to have nothing better to do than to extract the individual healing compounds from plants and sell them in the form of synthetic designer pills at the highest possible price. Why do they do it? Because one has the right to patent synthetic chemical compounds and earn a lot of money with them over a very long time. In many cases, valuable plants are being purchased by rogue companies who are buying sole rights to many indigenous and exotic plants worldwide, from corrupt governments.

Only Mother Nature knows how to bear plants with a perfect diversity and harmony of substances. Nothing is as effective as the natural, organic interaction of substances in a natural, healthy plant. Of course, modern pharmaceuticals also make use of herbs and plants, but mostly only extracts. The wisdom of nature cannot be copied. No laboratory can emulate nature. And we know that carnivorous animals also eat grasses and herbs from time to time for functional digestion. Animals still have this instinct, only we humans have lost it.

No wonder most pharmaceutical products don't effect a real healing! What they do manage very well is to cause side effects, which have to be 'treated' with even more pills. Clever economics, don't you think?

Cheap dietary supplements are also not good for our bodies. It has been shown in countless studies that cheap preparations are bad for the body and serve only to ease a bad conscience. Preparations which are supposed to deliver trace elements like iron, selenium, zinc, iodine, copper, manganese, molybdenum, chromium etc. usually offer them in far too high amounts, and they don't necessarily come from healthy agriculture.

These elements only exist in small traces in our bodies. The intake through normal nutrition and greens rich in minerals is usually sufficient for the body especially if one takes care with how one cooks them.

Sadly, there aren't as many plants rich in minerals anymore, due to bad agriculture practices which further cause poor soil conditions. One therefore needs to make an extra effort to seek out higher quality foods and supplements. I used supplementary products from the company LIFE. They were absolutely necessary for me, as 'help' with my seriously ill and exhausted body.

We humans are able to regenerate our bodies on a cellular level in an amazing way with plant- based diets, where the medical industry and doctors can only watch dumb from the sides. Modern medicine has certainly achieved much and performs extremely well in many areas such as in the case of emergencies. But when it comes to chronic diseases they mostly stand on lost ground.

Chlorophyll, for example, is one of the most researched substances. It is the green of the plant due to the process of converting sunlight into energy. Exactly how this transformation takes place has never been clarified in absolute detail. And yet it has also been recognised scientifically as an antiseptic agent and has historically been used for wound care. But it also has a variety of other healing qualities and uses. The watermelon is a very good chlorophyll donor.

Other 'all-rounders' include **chlorella** and **spirulina**. These are both algae rich in chlorophyll. Both contain vitamin B12 and are a good natural source for vegans.

Furthermore, studies have shown that chlorella is able to bind and remove heavy metals if consumed in the right way. Heavy metals such as lead, cadmium and mercury have a very harmful effect on our nervous system.

The above includes some of the most important nutrition principals that I derived through trial and error, and which have ultimately helped me overcome my MS disease significantly. On my **bonus resources** page you can find a link to a website with references to my daily routine, which may be of help.

CHAPTER 7: VITAMIN D3 – THE SUN HORMONE!

Vitamin D3 – the 'mains switch' of our body's functions
Vitamin D3 is sometimes called the sun-vitamin. In truth it's not a vitamin, rather it's a secosteroid hormone. **This vitamin primarily regulates the body's healing power**. Vitamin D3 is produced as a hormone when the skin is exposed to sunlight. Like the mains switch in your house, it regulates important processes in the body. When the vitamin D3 level is too low then the metabolic processes slow down. The body then thinks it has entered a period of reduction, as happens in winter, and it tries to build up its fat reserves as storage for harder times. Clearly, once vitamin D3 has been depleted in the body, losing weight is much harder than normal.

Many people in the northern countries suffer from vitamin D3 depletion. This is because the sun reaches the necessary intensity only from May to September. The book by Jeff T. Bowles, ***'The Miraculous Results Of Extremely High Doses Of The Sunshine Hormone Vitamin D3, My Experiment With Huge Doses Of D3 From 25,000 To 50,000 To 100,00 Iu A Day Over A 1 Year Period'***, describes very simply how vitamin D3, amongst other activities, regulates our endogenous 'repair - mechanisms'. If there is a lack of vitamin D3 then certain necessary 'repairs' don't take place in the body. Each cell in the body has a vitamin D3 receptor, so the level of vitamin D3 in the body directly affects all the cells. When D3 is depleted, our body is kept going on the barest minimum energy. But apart from that not much else can take place.

The sun as a vitamin D3 source

In Austria the average vitamin D3 level in the blood is about 8 – 12 ng/mL in winter, and about 18 – 25 ng/mL in summer. However, values below 20 ng/mL are regarded as a serious deficiency! From October to April it's not possible to build up vitamin D3 directly from sun shine because the angle of the sun causes the UVB rays to be filtered through the atmosphere. During these months we diminish our store of vitamin D3 and can slide from adequate to seriously deficient very rapidly. In other words, our skin produces vital vitamin D3 only during the summer when the sun's rays are at an optimal angle (and there is no presence of commercial sun protection cream).

But whoever believes he is doing his body a favour by 'roasting' in the sun for hours without protection is mistaken. The skin produces vitamin D3 with UVB radiation only in the first 10 - 15 minutes (according to skin type). This D3 is removed by UVA radiation, followed by skin damage through too long exposure to the sun. For your information, UVB radiation doesn't penetrate through window glass, whereas UVA radiation does. It is therefore impossible to get sunburn through a closed window.

How I came to high concentrate dosages of vitamin D3

It is best to have your blood tested for vitamin D3 by a doctor. Then you can decide what to do. I started independently with a daily dose of 100,000 IU (short for 'international units') in the form of drops, which is very concentrated, over a period of three months. I showed significant progress and slowly reduced the daily amount to 80,000 IU. Today I take a daily dose of 20,000 IU vitamin D3.

Besides the vitamin D3 drops I take vitamin K2 for protection, because vitamin D3 in high doses can reduce vitamin K2 levels in the body. Among other functions, vitamin K2 is responsible for storing calcium in the bones. For every 10,000 IU of Vitamin D3 I took one pill of vitamin K2 to be safe. At this point I want to emphasise that I only refer to my own personal xperiences in this book, and that I make **NO** therapeutic claims or suggestions whatsoever.

When I started taking the vitamin D3 in high dosages I combined it with large amounts of 'Oleovit D3' which is available in all Austrian pharmacies. The bottles contain 12.5 mL each (180,000 IU) which is only 400 IU per drop. Taking a daily dose of 80,000 IU I needed one flask every two days. I had to plan this carefully as Vitamin D3 preparations are only available on prescription in Austria, and the stipulation is only one bottle per store.

I sometimes needed the whole day to drive to all the pharmacies I knew to order enough vitamin D3. Driving around the streets to get my vital vitamin D3 made me feel like a drug addict. Naturally, this was no long-term solution so I started ordering vitamin D3 and K2 on the internet. Take note: It wasn't long before I noticed a big difference in quality. Generally, vitamin D3 and vitamin K2 products supplied by the more serious internet stores were not only higher in quality and concentration, but also much cheaper. I had to go to all this effort for a medication which relieved my illness and helped my fight to getting healthy again, which was not freely available at pharmacies in my country. Vitamin D3 is available without prescription in other countries like the USA, Italy and the Netherlands.

I once met some people on whom vitamin D3 therapy had no positive effect. This can apparently happen, and may be caused by the following: For people with damaged intestines, the absorption of vitamin D3 in the form of drops might be hindered or even totally blocked. Generally, people are not aware that they have a problem with their intestines. Such problems can remain unnoticed for a long time. One can live apparently problem-free for years but it will appear sooner or later. They have to explore other options such as sun studios with appropriate UVB lights, injections or regular sun bathing. Over time I was able to figure out the cause for bad absorption of vitamin D3 for everyone I know.

Vitamin D3 didn't only help with my MS, it also stimulated the circulations in my right hand. My arm and feet were always cold and numb. Both symptoms disappeared shortly after starting with the vitamin D3. Furthermore, after a short time I was able to pass two kidney stones **without pain** and without the very painful renal colic.

There are many researchers and doctors worldwide who have had success with high dosage vitamin D3 therapy. One example is Cicero G. Coimbra, MD, from Brazil, who reports success rates of up to 95%.

I would also recommend the book, *'Healthy in seven days – Success through Vitamin D treatment'*, by Raimund von Helden, MD. This book explains in detail how and why vitamin D3 has to be taken. You can find this and other books on my must-read booklist through the link on the **bonus resources** page.

CHAPTER 8: THE MOST IMPORTANT THING OF ALL IS WATER!

One can write a library of books on the single topic of water! Books by **F. Badmanghelidj MD** are all very informative and instructive. I can especially recommend *'Water Cures, Drugs Kill: How Water Cured Incurable Diseases'* (see bonus resources). This book relates success stories from people suffering with chronic diseases, and how their health improved radically through drinking water. It is a really encouraging book for those of you who think there is no more hope. I have read several books by F. Badmanghelidj MD and they were all good.

I drink at least 3 litres of water each day. Wasser is THE medicine par excellence. The human body is approximately 75 % water – more accurately said: 65 % oxygen and 10 % hydrogen, being 75 %. If one considers this composition it is quite clear that water is the most vital substance for a healthy body.

Each cell – and we all have 70 – 100 billion in us, is surrounded by water. This is referred to as lymphatic fluid. Via this lymphatic fluid all nutrients are delivered to our cells on the one hand, and on the other hand all by-products are removed. This represents our metabolism. If this fluid is unclean due to waste deposits and acids, our metabolism gets sluggish and the waste starts to decompose. All metabolic processes need a certain alkalinity to function healthily.

We need acids as well, but everything should be in a healthy balance. The human pH value is between 7.35 and 7.45 and thus slightly alkaline.

For the body to survive it is essential to maintain a blood pH value level of between 6.8 and 8. If this wasn't the case, even for just a few seconds, we would immediately die. The pH value is kept constant by the lungs and kidneys.

The pH scale goes from 1 to 14. A pH value of more than 7 (7 – 14) is called alkaline. A pH value below 7 (1 – 7) is called acidic.

The expression pH originates from Latin and means 'potentia hydrogenii' (potency of hydrogen). If the lymph fluid is polluted, or worse, too 'dehydrated', then this can lead to a variety of major health problems. Dehydration is very common in our society. Most people think that if they just drink colas, coffee or alcohol, or sweetened beverages, that they will have enough fluids in their bodies. They justify this by saying, "But I already drank one litre of juice." This is a misconception.

It has been proven that by drinking just one litre of juice, more fluid is *removed* from the body through urine and the skin than what was previously consumed. Consider classic coffee culture: In all coffee shops (at least in Austria), you will be served a glass of water with your coffee order. Why? To clean and replenish the fluids of the body! This is because coffee and tea are strong diuretics (have a tendency to increase the discharge of urine). Apart from sugar, most drinks and juices contain additives to control flavour and extend shelf life. These artificial additives cannot be processed by the body; they are a burden to the body and have to be disposed of. In order to rinse out and dispose of these poisons the body needs clean water.

If there is no clean water, or insufficient water, then this process can't take place and so the body becomes toxic. Toxins can only be removed with the intake of clean water. But how can this take place if the only liquids consumed are already polluted and toxic before they enter the body? Anyone who has tried to clean the floor with dirty water knows what I am talking about. When one calculates the accumulation of pollutants and toxins in the body one can understand how eventually the body dehydrates and illnesses set in. In dehydrated conditions even the blood becomes sluggish and this is certainly life-threatening. In order to avoid this, the blood takes water from the lymphatic fluids and so a vicious cycle sets in which leads to further health complications.

Ultimately, it is hardly possible to support a normal, healthy metabolism when the fluids in the body are full of waste and toxins. How can dirty, dehydrated blood and fluids transport oxygen and nutrients to the cells? It can't. So all the slag and waste stays in the body. This is how many diseases start. To top it, the very medicine we take to cure the illness gets stuck in this brew and can't help us. Everything which gets stuck in this brew turns acidic, feeding the downward spiral.

Let's think about an aquarium: we regularly test the water and remove algae from the glass. We nurture our fish with the best nutrients and hygiene measures in order to maintain a healthy environment, for healthy fish. Unfortunately, we don't care as much for our own bodies. We become ill and wonder why.

Drinking water heals – without water nothing is possible!

It is advisable to drink alkaline purified water e.g. filtered water. If it is not available then normal tap water will do. Water helps to neutralize the surplus acids within us. It is important to avoid water that comes through old lead water pipes. Fungi and cancers favour an acidic milieu. There are a variety of diseases which can be avoided by drinking enough water.

But not all water is the same! Mineral water, whether carbonated or still, is not suitable to 'clean' the body. Mineral water, as the name suggests, contains minerals, but our body needs water without minerals. Why? Because the water is needed for carrying our own nutrition or waste, which it can't do it if the water is already saturated. It's like not being able to get onto the train because it is already packed with passengers. I know that very well from Vienna.

A word on fungi in the body
While speaking of water I would like to mention something here. Wherever there is water, **fungi** are not far. And where there are fungi – in or on the body – something is wrong. On our skin we have a lot of fungi which, on a normally healthy body, causes no damage. But if the fungi spreads aggressively e.g. in our intestines or on our skin, we have more than just a fungi problem. A fungus is always a sign that something is out of balance and has to be 'recycled'. In this case it's we ourselves that have to do the work. That may sound funny, but it isn't. Humidity, bad hygiene, heat and acidity create the ideal conditions for fungi. If the breeding ground (our fluid system) is cleaned up, then the fungi will disappear of its own accord.

A simple comparison is a house full of fungal infestations. A fungicide may destroy the fungi in one area, but in reality the fungus hasn't disappeared completely and it is likely to flare up again in a different spot. The only way to get rid of the fungus altogether is to dry out and sanitise the walls of the house. Only then will the fungus disappear.

Regardless of whether the fungi is internal or external, if one 'starves' the breeding ground of the fungi it will disappear by itself. Pills, whether chemical or natural, may eliminate the fungi from its current site, but it will just as soon appear elsewhere. This game will last for as long as it takes the body to cleanse itself and regain a healthy balance, in which case there are no more 'recycling tasks' left for the fungi.

CHAPTER 9: ELIMINATION AND DETOXIFICATION

The topic of digestion and elimination is extremely important because everything we take into our bodies needs to be absorbed, and the waste or by-products properly removed. This cycle has to happen in the right way if we are to maintain good health.

The various nutrients of what we consume are distributed throughout the body. The waste is then carried via the lymphatic system and removed from the body via the intestines, the lungs, the kidneys and the skin. These are our four primary waste disposal systems. Alternative practitioner, Gunther Wolfgang Schneider, wrote an excellent book with the title '*Biotop Mensch – Liebe Deine Darmbakterien – Paradigmenwechsel in der Medizin*' **(Organic man – Love your enterobacteria – a Paradigm shift in medicine only available in German).**

The intestines and our health

The intestine and its mucous membranes as well as the intestinal flora, play a very important role. Many people suffer from intestine, colon and digestion problems as I do. I am still working at trying to bring everything into balance again. Irrespective of whether one suffers from diarrhoea or constipation, ultimately everything has the same origin: the body is too acidic.

Each person's bowels react differently. In one person the bowels hold back while in another it tries to eliminate as quickly as possible. In order to process and eliminate correctly, our intestines need billions of special bacteria. We cannot live without these good bacteria!

If the intestinal flora changes because the body has become too acidic, then the mucous membranes and all the good bacteria are negatively affected, which causes good bacteria and harmless fungi to turn aggressive.

Simply put, this means that the intestine is not able to fully absorb, in a normal and healthy way, the nutrition supplied to it. This means that the more important nutrients do not reach the cells. In this case even the best and healthiest foods cannot nourish the body. To top it all, the undigested substances, which remain in the intestines, increase the acidity level of the body as they ferment and rot before being eliminated. At some point, our body tells us that something is going badly wrong, and we get sick.

Did you know that with harmonious intestinal flora toilet paper wouldn't be necessary? There is a very simple and safe test which anyone can do at home: After your next bowel movement, try to observe if the stool is covered in a form of mucous membrane. If it is there should be no 'smudges' in the toilet, and the cleaning of your rear wouldn't be necessary. Healthy stools leave no trace. If our stool does, then we know there could be a problem.

A **sick intestine** can make us ill as 80% of our immune system is controlled in the intestines. I find it strange that people with intestinal ailments and diseases don't give a thought as to where it might originate. Some say its destiny and some blame it on bad genes. Perhaps it's a bit of both. But it is really very simple. We need to realise that everything we consume has to be processed, absorbed by the body and the waste excreted.

If I fill my body with junk food, harmful foods (frozen, artificial etc) and sweetened liquids, it will burden the intestines, and inflammations and cancers may result.

I need a target, and the will to make a change

Healthy nutrition can prevent a lot of diseases. I changed my nutrition but it wasn't easy at the beginning. What's important is that we change our thinking and our awareness. Of course I loved huge burgers and roast pork. Cola was my favourite drink. So it took me some to recognise and come to terms with the wealth of fruit and vegetables, before I was able to give up my old ways. For a tasty meat substitute I discovered granulated soy. I once served it to guests as spaghetti sauce and nobody recognised it was made without meat. One thing is clear: I first have to want to change and have a goal in mind, and then nothing can come in my way!

The skin as excretory organ

The skin is our largest excretory organ, and is closely linked to the intestines. If the intestines are ill, the skin is also ill. If the intestines are not able to remove all the accumulated waste, then the skin has to step in. We exhale toxins, so to speak, via our skin. The stronger the odour of our perspiration, the more toxic the substances are that are being removed through the skin. Every eczema on our skin is a sign that the intestines are no longer able to process all the toxins, which means they must be removed through the skin. No matter which medication we use to treat our eczema it will come back as long as we have a clogged and ailing intestine that needs to be cleansed.

But the skin has got a more important function - it breathes. And through it oxygen is transported to the lungs.

There, oxygen molecules enter the red blood cells which then transport them throughout the body. If the skin is overworked by detoxifying you, it isn't able to fulfil this second, important function in the right way. But in order to survive, cells need oxygen otherwise they suffocate and turn cancerous. Only a cell which doesn't get oxygen can turn cancerous. And then we have a really big problem.

Scrutinizing the relationships in our body

Obviously, every part of our body is interconnected. A blockage in any vital cycle or process is very likely to impair our health. The intestines have to function in the right way for the healthy absorption of nutrients and the removal of pollutants. The skin has to be able to breathe in order to absorb oxygen for the cells. A malfunction in any of these fundamental processes hinders the functioning of other processes and organs such as delivery via the blood, the metabolism via the lymphatic fluid, the excretion of toxic substances and the retention of vital minerals in/from our connective tissue and bones. If nothing can flow due to toxins and blockages then our cells start to suffocate or malnourish and become ill.

With time our blood may turn viscous and sluggish as a consequence of dehydration and pollution, and then it can no longer pass through the small capillaries. This causes the circulatory disturbances which many of us know too well. If a blockage happens in the veins it can cause phlebitis, or even a thrombosis. If such a 'plug' releases itself, it may lead to a life-threatening heart attack, stroke or pulmonary infarction.

I don't need any of that anymore! I already have a very full rucksack to carry. Although even in my case body fluidity was an issue.

Because of the inactivity of my legs and my right arm, my body accumulated lymphatic fluid, and I had to tackle the problem fast. I still have problems with it but only in the one leg and in my right arm. Although I now know how to regulate it and remain below danger level.

The blockage of lymphatic fluid such as I suffered from is treated in two different ways: Either through lymphatic drainage by a physiotherapist, or through movement. I decreased the blockage through a lot of movement and massaging myself, because I couldn't afford a physiotherapist. I realised that a lot of things were possible even without having a lot of money. Don't be discouraged and give up if you have a limited budget. Become inventive. Be creative. By searching for alternatives and solutions one often gets along with much less, or no money at all. For example, you can buy yourself a 'hedgehog ball'. With such a ball you can easily massage the relevant areas yourself to promote lymph activity.

The kidneys and their limits
They kidneys are the next in our removal- and detoxing cycle. They have the task of functioning as filters. They filter out all the minerals and other nutrients from the 'waste water' in our bodies. The rest is removed from the body as urine. As I said previously, I drink a lot of water which helps to remove the redundant waste. Part of my self - training was to banish my pee bottle. It used to stand near my bed out of reach, which forced me to get up. That really helped to strengthen my body. As I mentioned, everything has the potential to become a training tool! Don't ever give up on yourself. There is a lot more in you than you might think. You just don't know it yet!

Waste and acids which can't be removed from tired, overworked intestines also end up in the kidneys, which will then have an even heavier workload than normal. Drinking water helps the kidneys to do their job.

The kidneys clean our blood. They are very diligent and manage to clean between 150 and 200 litres per day. But not more. This cleaning up means flushing out all the unwanted substances and transporting it via the water you drink to the bladder to pass as urine. Simply explained, our kidneys can't tolerate acidic blood and fluids over long periods. They get tired and become sluggish. If the kidneys are constantly overworked they become weak, which may well lead to dialysis or even kidney failure, in which case a kidney transplant will be required. Please don't get me wrong, my explanations are put very simply so that everyone can understand. I acknowledge fully that all the processes within the body are a lot more complicated and intricate than my basic descriptions here.

Beyond the lungs

Our lungs are another important organ for the removal of toxins from the body. Everybody knows that we inhale oxygen from the air and exhale carbon dioxide (CO_2). If we were not able to exhale the surplus CO_2, we would die very quickly. We would suffocate from the accumulation of CO_2 which would subsequently prevent the intake of new oxygen. We exhale everything our lungs turn into a gas which is harmful for us.

Smoking is the most damaging habit for the lungs. A smoker does not only have to process and remove all the 'normal' environmental pollutants as does everyone else, but also the highly toxic content of the cigarettes.

I enjoyed this vice too once, but soon recognised that smoking was not for me. It harms one on many levels and to boot it costs a fortune. But that's common knowledge.

The psychological and habit-forming effects from smoking are also very dangerous since nicotine has the capacity to overcome the blood-brain-barrier in seconds.

Less known is that the negative effects of smoking are not limited to the lungs. It spreads through the tissues into the lymphatic system and further afield to the cells. There the nicotine molecules stick, amongst others, onto cell receptors, which are in turn responsible for the absorption of nutrients. If the cell is no longer able to absorb nutrients because the receptors are contaminated by nicotine, it literally starves to death despite the offer of a full meal. Thus smoking affects the whole body not only the lungs and brain.

Nutrition and detox - a conclusion
What I described above became for me the most important principles of nutrition and elimination. I studied the theories, and combined these with precise planning and implementation with the purpose of recovering from this illness. Truly, there stretches a long road behind me full of trials and errors. Some things helped while others didn't. I tried to be cautious and use my common sense. Sometimes I made rather rash decisions because I almost felt I didn't have much to lose.

As mentioned above, good nutrition is vital for good health and recovery.

But in the beginning, even an excellent diet of clean and healthy foods may not help immediately, if the excretory organs are so worn and burdened that they are not able to absorb and transport the nutrients.

Everything I apply today, I have worked very hard for. It's not plain theory; it comes from my own trials, efforts and observations. I am no expert on the topic but even my mistakes had certain positive aspects that I am very grateful for. That is why I share these principles as vivid, practical examples for you to try out yourself. Please play with the ideas and experiment for yourself. Inform yourself sufficiently and act in a responsible way towards your body. It was my life I was dealing with. And now it's about yours.

Nutrition and detoxification are very important first elements to regaining and retaining our health. In my **bonus resources** page you will find more information.

CHAPTER 10: OUR THOUGHTS

Thoughts are life-determining!
Everything we think determines our life!

For years I have pondered the fascinating subject of thinking. I have read many books, talked with various people and observed their behaviour. I recommend books by **Alice Miller** to everyone who wants to experience and learn more about himself. You will have many 'wow-moments' and learn much about yourself, your behaviour and your chosen way of life. I read all the books by Alice Miller and they changed my life.

We all have one thing in common: **Our thoughts determine our lives!** I am neither a psychologist, nor do I have any official education in that area, but I have a clear and alert mind and I observe things.

Are we able to change ourselves?
I once worked as a pest controller. In this capacity of 'saviour' against unwanted pests, one gets to know people and their private world quite well. When people are afraid you see their real face. I don't wish to pass any opinions or create any theories on this, I simply with to share from my own experiences, observations, and from the gut-feel wisdom that resulted from it. During this time I got to know different characters, or life attitudes; calculating, brave, hysterical, fearful, daring, crazy, cautious, etc. They lived, acted and thought exactly in accordance with their basic 'life attitude'. Such strong characteristics, with all the thoughts and feelings that go with them, deep in the being of the person, are difficult to hide. Even more difficult to change.

Of course one could avoid looking at it by saying, "I am like I am", or "I've always been this way" or "I was born this way so I can't change". Even then, when I saw through my customers' masks, I thought it was normal and that everyone was like them and that one could not change.

But it isn't true. Every one of us WAS "made this way"!

How does our environment shape our thoughts and behaviour?

You may well ask how we were 'made this way'. The answer is: Through our education and our environment. Each person is born with the same attitudes; free from prejudices and judgement of our environment. Our parents are the ones who 'educate' us and impart us with THEIR adult view of the world. Furthermore our relatives, friends, teachers, bosses etc add to this 'education'. This wealth of information helps to form us into what we eventually become. And if there are no really radical experiences or crisis in our lives, then we usually just stay like that, unchanged.

It's often exactly the 'radical experience' that provides us with a more real and deeper insight into ourselves, into our true I. Sometimes these insights are so significant that they inspire us to change our lives dramatically and give us a shove in a new direction. These radical experiences might be a trauma or life threatening disease, the loss of a loved one or an accident etc. Whatever it is, without such events we may not be willing or able to make significant change in our lives.

Our character and behaviour are formed to some extent by our environment. Out of this our thoughts are created and as a result our deeds and actions. The bottom line is that everybody decides for himself how he wants to act, whether to do something or not, to be honest or not. The sum of intentions, in combination with our actions, ultimately forms our real character.

What about our trained behaviours and thought patterns? How have we 'learned' to lead our lives? Have we have allowed ourselves to become dependent on miscellaneous addictions like smoking, criticism, TV, alcohol or drugs to feel good? Do we rely on beverages, fast food and other quick meals for daily nutrition? Then we are heading straight for physical disaster.

These habits are often strengthened by excuses like we don't have time to cook a 'healthy' meal, because everything has to happen quickly. Permanent, excessive stress is seen today as normal. Then for relaxation we turn to a quick cigarette and a cup of coffee. Oh yes, we even don't have time to sleep, because during this time something exciting could happen which we don't want to miss like a movie on TV, an email or newscast. For security we put our cell phones next to our beds in order to be ready round the clock in case we might actually fall asleep.

What doesn't change is the fact that such a detrimental lifestyle makes us ill. When the disease eventually hits, it's a huge disaster. Then the only question is how big the disaster is. Heart attack, stroke, cancer, or even an allergy, rheumatism, gout, or an autoimmune disease. Pick any one of them. Which one would you rather have?

Each of them will restrict your life dramatically. It will not only restrict your life, it may change it completely.

How you can change your thinking and your behaviour
If one doesn't respond to the stress warnings and signals our body gives us, it will continue until it is forced to give up. Sooner or later it will have to, if the level of suffering is too high. Our body is a gift from nature, from the earth, and we can choose our attitude towards it. We don't need to be clever scientists to recognise when something is wrong with us, and to make our own choices on how to act.

I wrote this book for all those who may be touched, and for those of you who may not have been willing to walk this path in the first place. I have a bad disease. Multiple sclerosis is a disease which no one would like to have. I speak from my own painful experience when I say,
"Let's change it, before it forces us to change!"

Each of us, even you, has to deal with the question of whether or not you want to get rid of harmful old patterns. Do we want to develop further as human beings? Do we want to get rid of habits and behaviour patterns that are harmful for us? Through a sincere listening to yourself, deep within, we can sense whether we want to live the life we have or not; was it consciously chosen or is it a taught or implanted behaviour?

Our subconscious mind is home to various behavioural patterns and dogmas of which we are mostly not aware. If we pull them out of our subconscious mind we may find them to be much more disturbing than we thought.

Certainly, they are neither healthy nor helpful. Sometimes we know something is wrong or not in harmony with us, and although we might understand it to some degree, we are still not able to change it due to being held back by one or another of these unconscious dogmas or attitudes. Try to recognise them. NOW is always a good time to start. Get rid of those old thoughts and wrong patterns. They simply hinder us.

If we want to grow and change consciously, towards being free human beings, then exactly those automatic thoughts and deeds are our greatest hindrance. If we develop consciously we remain awake and connected at each step, each crisis, and then we start to take responsibility for ourselves. Once we do this we make a commitment to ourselves which requires enormous courage. Yes, we do need a big dose of courage to live the truth, and to make our lives that important. We have been taught to do the exact opposite: toe the line, do as you are told, don't make waves, don't change the status quo, everyone else must come first, not you.

But do we really subscribe to this? What about our individual characters and biographies? Are we happy to be one of the in-crowd? Or always the last one in line? I don't mean the obvious egotists, rather those who have unlearned to take responsibility by allowing themselves to be determined by outside forces, or have succumbed to their own automatic, unconscious behaviours. I speak about a healthy egoism, about joy and a love for one's self, not only others. We have mostly been taught to sacrifice ourselves for whatever greater good, and for others – our family, wife, children, parents, etc.

Over the years old thinking patterns remove us from our true I. We get more and more unhappy, bitter, tired or grumpy. Then we try to fill up this inner emptiness with consumer goods which we don't need. Or we eat excessively or distract ourselves with some triviality in order to avoid feeling and dealing with the pain within.

When we take back responsibility for ourselves, and find the courage to live in truth, we may feel as if we have arrived 'home' again, in ourselves, and we may finally uncover our true self, without bitterness or resentment. Then we may experience a sense of joy and especially gratitude towards ourselves. In this positive state we are able to nourish that space within, to warm it and bring it joy.

All our thoughts are transformed into energy. Do we constantly feel empty? Bitter or tired? In that case diseases have an easy task. Now is the time to change. Consider seriously that our words, thoughts and feelings form our reality. There is a very wise saying which I once read,

'There are people with the opinion, that certain problems and conflicts can't be solved.
These people are right for two reasons:
Firstly, because the world is what each person thinks it is.
And secondly, because many problems are actually not solvable with conventional thinking.'

CHAPTER 11: DEATH AND IMMORTAL LIFE

The impulse that set me on the path out of darkness and released me from 'hell', was my confrontation with death. I know this subject is taboo for many people. Nevertheless, I believe it important to raise the subject and discuss it here, even if just briefly.

The fear of dying and getting healthy

Many people are afraid to die and this fear blocks our life energy. This anxiety is deeply rooted in the conscious as well as the subconscious mind. It is very important to free oneself from this fear because only then are we open and free to live fully. This anxiety also prevents us from letting go of all that old 'stuff', which hinders new things coming into our lives. It is the same when it comes to healing. Actually, we are more often than not afraid of a change in our disease - we tend to hold onto the old because it is familiar and safe, and change may well bring something scary - the unknown.

We may well die while trying to change. We stay on the safe side with attitudes like, "The doctor said....", and we follow his advice like the good boys and girls we were taught to be in our childhood. Through our education we have 'unlearned' to take self-responsibility, or rather, it was taken away from us by that education. Very few people actually want to, or are even able to take responsibility for their own lives because of the paralyzing fear of death that lurks in the background. But we can re-learn to take responsibility and free ourselves from this fear. Dealing with our crisis consciously, with issues of death and our anxieties, liberates us so that our life energy can flow again, unhindered.

When we face our fears we become aware of our vulnerability and the reality of death. But thinking about it frighten us even more and so we continue to avoid it.

We can only heal ourselves if we cross our own borders, jump over our own shadows, and face those blocks and paralyzing anxieties of death.

Our birth came with an expiry date
As young, healthy people we don't want know anything about death. Being old and sick doesn't change this either. Most of us don't want to get to grips with death at any stage even though we were given an expiry date before we even arrived. Regardless of how; through accident, disease, suicide or even because our biological clock has run out, we will all have to cross the threshold to the other side sooner or later. And yes, every one of us has to make this special journey on his or her own, regardless of who is there with your body 'till the end'.

While living in the here and now we have a natural will to survive which is given to us by our development and evolution. This will to survive might change to some degree due to illness or emotional pain. But this will is also able to do something else: it is able to give us extraordinary strength, which we may only recognise under crisis or traumatic circumstances.

In my case, I didn't want to live any longer *with* my disease. But my will for life was unshaken. I asked myself, "Is this all there is to it? You are 46 years old, is that all there is to life?"

I had many conversations with myself and imagined that 'place over there on the other side'.

Is there such a place? I don't like the suggestions offered by religion. Religions make several claims that I can't comprehend or identify with in any way. Like many people I am too much of a realist. But I can't deny the existence of something simply because I don't see it or understand it. In principle I believe life is eternal, and I am actually able to explain this.

We all are made of cosmic atoms

I can deal with the fact that we are all made from innumerable atoms which have existed over billions of years. We are all made of stardust. Each atom within us was forged in a star. Only through its 'death' via a supernova were atoms released for use elsewhere.

Everything I say here has been scientifically proven. Our own sun consists of exactly the same atoms which we are made of. Each planet in our solar system was created with these atoms. Actually, all suns and their planets resulted from the supernova of other suns.

My point is that there is no death in reality because all matter is transformed and used elsewhere to create new life.

That our body has an expiry date doesn't mean the end. It is just a new beginning. This is the eternal cycle of nature. Physically we can't die because the atoms from which we were made are unbreakable, whether we are cremated or buried in the usual way. Atoms can only be changed through nuclear fusion or nuclear fission, but they can't be destroyed.

Consciousness energy

The question now arises as to what happens to our knowledge, our feelings, our will and consciousness? Albert Einstein once said that energy can neither disappear, nor is it destructible. Energy is matter. Science states that the energy which drives us to live can't disappear.

If our conscious energy doesn't disappear, where does it go? I want to show it plastically. If one blows out a burning candle, the flame might be dead and gone, but the energy is still in the room in the form of heat. The heat is no longer concentrated on the top of the wick, but spread into the room as residual heat. The bigger the room, the less we notice this heat around us. But it is always measurable as residual radiation.

Our consciousness doesn't disappear either. It just spreads around us. The earth is full of such energy. Each living being is surrounded by it.

Scientists have busied themselves throughout time with the mystery of exactly what it is that sparks the life in something, how life actually comes about. If a man and a woman unite life arises all by itself. An energy leaps over, unites itself and a new life begins. To this day science has not been able to bring something artificial to life. Nature, however, creates life constantly, billions of times each day.

What comes after death?

We all are born over and over again with a 'new' life, a new energy. There are numerous fascinating stories of reincarnation which one may or may not want to believe.

Time and time again, children are born with clear memories of a former life. They know details about people, their names, their residences as well as the 'life' itself which they used to live. Most of them are children who want to share the memories or ask questions. In all cases they had never visited any of the places in their current life. They only have the memories, and in many cases the accuracy of the stories were verified and proven to be correct through research and investigation. No one is able to explain this phenomenon. These children come from different religions and different regions all over the world. As I said before, you may believe it or not. At least a window of unexplored possibilities is opened through these stories. We are far away from knowing everything.

I find the idea of what might await us after our 'death' very exciting. Like everyone else, I have no idea what awaits me. But what I do know is that it will be exactly how it is meant to be, and that is good.

Generally we can't say exactly where we come from or where we are returning to. Let's imagine we would know who we were, or where we came from. Exactly this would frighten me - the knowledge of my body and my being transforming throughout time. The known universe has probably existed around 13.76 billion years. In all this time a kind of continual transformation of matter, of earth, of culture has taken place where out of the old, something new can arise.

If we automatically knew about our former lives, it would become boring in the sense that we may see everything as being predictable.

We may be angry or disappointed if we thought we didn't have the same chances as in a prior life and may wish to end our lives with the hope of a new and better beginning, like we are tempted to do in videogames where one has infinite lives in order to win a game. If things aren't going well for us we simply discard our player with the hope of getting a better one for the next round. How boring that would be in real life! One might even get a worse deal. There would be no challenge to confront hardship and grow. We would only experience the same thing over and over again. Like robots.

If we try to come to terms with all speculations, with all esoteric and religious concepts, we would become very confused with all the contradictions. I suggest we remain ignorant and be glad about it because then we can then experience every moment as an exciting challenge.

We need not be frightened of death. If we were constantly afraid of dying we wouldn't find the time to live fully.

Living in the present
We could all try to live in the here and now and not be afraid of our death which lies somewhere in the future. Instead, we could try to live more consciously and make the best out of every day and every single moment. Let's learn to enjoy our lives again, to appreciate our family, our friends, our common strivings, until we are called back for the next big adventure.

When was the last time we hugged, kissed or told our children or our partner that we loved them? When was the last time we laughed together and had fun with our friends?

When last did we go deeply into ourselves and praise and love ourselves for who we are? It is very important to accept and love ourselves just as we are. There is no one other than 'us' right now.

The first step to happiness and health is to be satisfied with ourselves and love ourselves as we are with all our strengths and weaknesses. If we manage to live in peace with ourselves and to accept our weaknesses, we may well be able to turn them into great insights and strengths.

CHAPTER 12: THE DVD WHICH CHANGED MY LIFE

On 20 March 2014 (soon after my new resolve) I watched a DVD by Helmuth Matzner which put me even further on the right path. My good friend, Christine, called me out of the blue and said, "I watched a DVD and you have to watch it too!" So I ordered it, and watched it together with Petra, my partner. I was very excited when I recognized the chance of losing weight by following their suggestions. I wanted to lose a lot of weight, but if there was a chance to improve my health at the same time I would certainly embrace it.

The DVD was about nutrition and how to get healthy by eating the right things. I didn't really consider my health at that stage as I was more excited at the prospect of losing weight, since at that stage I still weighed 108 kg!

As Petra and I finished watching the DVD I said, "Go to the refrigerator immediately and throw out all the useless food in it!" What do you think my good wife answered? She looked at me with big eyes and said "No, I won't do that! Are you crazy? All those things cost a lot of money and I won't throw it out!" Being a good husband I immediately accepted this argument. But after a minute or two I replied, "OK, in that case I will consume everything myself until it is empty, and then we will go out and buy only the good stuff." I didn't hesitate a moment longer and true to my word I consumed everything in the shortest possible time. From that moment on we only bought healthy, nutritious foods: bananas, apples, different kinds of salads, and so on….. sometimes I had no idea what we were actually buying!

Like always, Petra was my salvation. She bought things with names I might have heard at some point in my life but had never actually seen. Avocados, mangos, papayas, cress, soy granules and a lot more became our staple diet. Everything which she had been telling me but I never wanted to listen to. I would refer to it as 'her stuff' which she was always on about. Now she was in the position to say, "I told you so". And I had to admit, "Yes, you were right all the time, although bananas, which I always ate, are healthy too." I just had to save face a little.

My stubborn ego needed a rubdown now and again, but by now everything had changed. I looked in the internet for Helmuth Matzner's phone number and called him immediately. I wanted to arrange an appointment with him to learn more about good and right nutrition, and if there was any chance of me getting healthy again.

The first meeting
We arranged to meet Helmuth Matzner at one of his lectures a few days later. Petra and I drove to the appointment. She helped me to get from the car into the building, which meant that I had to walk about 30 m. At that stage, in order to walk at all, I needed to hold onto Petra with one hand and hold onto a walking stick with the other. The truth is that I didn't want to arrive there in a wheelchair. And so with Petra and walking stick I dragged myself through the entrance of the building, to the big hall. Mr Matzner recognised me immediately.

He knew that I had to be the man who was able to walk only with great effort. He even greeted me by my name, and this is how everything began.

I learned a lot from him about health. He gave me a lot of books to read which were a boost in the right direction. Among the many books he recommended was the book I mentioned previously about vitamin D3 which was unknown to me at that stage. He stressed that I had to read this special book very carefully as it may be of great help to me. I read the book and thought it worth a try.

Vitamin D3 - first drops

It took some time before I started with the vitamin D3 drops because at that stage I had a lot of books to read and the drops seemed to be less important. So it was only some weeks later that I received my order of drops and started my 'dangerous' experimenting with high dosages of vitamin D3. The author, Jeff T. Bowles, called his own self-experiment with vitamin D3 'dangerous' (but also with inverted commas).

The vitamin D3 drops started working immediately and accelerated my self-healing power to such a degree that I was almost free of pain after only a couple of days. I hardly believed it. In fact, I had almost no pain at all when walking, lying or moving my arms or legs. This freedom from pain completely convinced me about the effectiveness of the high dosage vitamin D3 treatment.

About my diary records

In the next chapter I would like to share some of my diary entries. They tell my story in a much more exciting and concise way than if I was to summarise it all. I will quote from relevant texts and elaborate on them.

Furthermore, at the end of the book there is a **bonus resources** page with links to an exclusive website for my readers, where you can learn more about my background and history as well as the resources and tools which helped me. There you will also find audio visual material on the various situations as described in my diary entries.

CHAPTER 13: EXTRACTS FROM MY DIARY

Diary entries

Note: I filmed some short videos exclusively for readers of this book. They show the actual locations and settings described in some of my diary entries. Further down you will find the link to these videos on my **bonus resources** page.

1 January 2014: Today is the start of my third life. I don't know where this new road will lead me but anywhere is better than wasting away and dying slowly. I will think of nothing other than how to become healthy again. I am 46 years old and I want to live with dignity or die fast. I don't know which lessons I need to learn this lifetime, but if something or someone truly exists up there then please don't get in my way. I, myself, will decide about my own life so stay away from me or help me. I want to participate in and enjoy life actively again. The first thing I want to do is lose weight. I weigh 110 kg. I want to change something in my life.

I had no idea at this stage how much would eventually change.

12 January 2014: Every morning I suffer from severe convulsions and spasms. They start even if Petra touches me very softly. It is extremely painful but I don't dare to take more than 125 mg Lioresal and 48 mg Hydal. It is hard for me to get out of bed and after a walk to the bathroom I am both exhausted and tired. I get up 10 times a day on purpose so that my muscles remain active.

I lean on the bed for as long as I can endure it and then sit down again. I do this at least 10 times a day. Today I managed it 15 times. It's just like it was at the fitness centre in the early days, only much shorter.

I almost got used to the pain because if one has extreme pain for long enough periods of time, one can become resistant or numbed to it in some way. I became less sensitive to my pain. Sure it hurt, but in a different way. It is hard to describe, one develops something of a thick skin. Today I didn't take either a painkiller or Lioresal because I have gotten rid of my spasms, convulsions and pain. Thank heavens, so to speak. Just thinking back now on how hard it was for me in the beginning to simply stand up, and how naturally I do it today, I only can say Awesome! Today I am able to train again with my bar-bells and re-build my lost muscles.

20 January 2014: This morning I was able to get up and stand immediately. I had to steady my wobbling by bending my knees a little but it felt good. Spasms and convulsions have gotten stronger because of the training sessions. I think this is because everything is bit inflamed with the exercise. My right hand is cold and stiff even though I put it into warm water and rubbed it.

Just don't get frightened in the beginning. At first things do get worse, but then they get better. It may simply be that your body isn't used to it anymore. Muscle cramps and weaknesses are normal in the beginning. Just keep going and success will come on its own. It just needs a bit of time. Perhaps one could reduce the training a little but don't give up training altogether.

If one suffers from cold hands or feet then a warm bath will help, even if only for a short time, but it's better than nothing.

2 February 2014: Its one month later, I have been working my ass off and have hardly noticed a change. Standing and walking still hurts but I did manage once to stand up 30 times. I am able to stand for 3 minutes, but then I can´t continue. I read a lot and try to learn new things, but reading is very exhausting for me. My eyes only see sharply at a distance of 40-50 cm. I watched the DVD from Bruce Lipton at least 10 times, but I just don't get it. Am I too stupid for it? I meditate and practice Yoga as best as I can.

At the beginning it takes a really long time to get your body going. I lay in bed and did nothing for a very long time and so everything is difficult and twice as exhausting. Breaks are very important while training and building the body up. To work out every day might not be a good idea, although one should do something for the body every day. But it is important to vary it. I do strength training on one day and then take a break for at least three days. The body needs time to recover and build up. Yoga and stretching is a good workout for every day but be careful not to overextend yourself. I do endurance training three times a week. I can fully understand if it is hard for you in the beginning, but don't give up. Or do you have something else to do besides getting healthy?! Every time I took a break I read, did research and made sure I learned something new. I read everything that could possibly help me to get healthy again. Use the time between your training sessions wisely to learn something new. It is never too late to learn new stuff.

17 February 2014: Today I started taking Magnesium for my convulsions. I wanted to see if it helped. I noticed that while standing I had more endurance, but my hips and sacrum soon got weak and I had to lie down afterwards. Then I needed two hours to get back on my feet again. I stand up very consciously now and bend my knees until I can't anymore. I managed to get up 18 times in two hours. With Petra on one arm and a walking stick in my other hand, I was able to walk about 40 m!

Later I noticed that there is Magnesium, and there is Magnesium! Each mineral or vitamin needs to be an organic substance or it may not help. Sadly, it would seem that industries don't care how they mix their minerals because many of the dietary supplements and multivitamins on offer do not help at all. I think this says something of the 'system' behind it because, even if it helps just a little, the customer will buy more and more in his efforts to cure his illness. Well, that's also an option.

04 March 2014: Two months of torture are lying behind me. My right arm and hand are still numb, stiff and cold. It doesn't matter what I try, it stays numb and cold. In order to warm it I lie on it. The pressure feels good but it doesn't improve it at all. The whole arm remains useless. Getting up has become a meditation and it works quite well. I don't count how often I do it anymore because I am now able to do it well and often. Only the spasms and convulsions continue to torture me. I can walk with assistance for 50 m. Magnesium doesn't help although I take it every day.

Even after two months I didn't give up because I have a strong dream.

And it is very important that you create a strong dream for yourself too. And I have already had one success: I was able to stand up uncountable times, because I repeated it so often. And therein lies a secret. The magical word is 'repetition'. Repeat it so often that it becomes normal. Do not give up; start over and over again!

20 March 2014: Watched the DVD with Petra. Unlike her I was excited. I saw enrichment where she could only see abstinence. It was as if the scales fell from my eyes. It became obvious to me what I actually do the whole time. What a big difference! Here is a new task, something new for me to do which gives me hope and a new impulse for my life. Empty the refrigerator by eating everything in it and buy fresh healthy food. The changeover is easy: just replace unhealthy food with healthy food. I weigh 108 kg now and my goal weight is 80 kg!!!

You have to consider the fact that your own partner may not share your opinions. Don't let yourself be irritated by relatives or friends. It's YOUR life that counts. Whether your partner has the same diet as you or not, is not important. You can eat your food and your partner can eat his or hers. Petra still eats things from time to time which I don't. You only have to resist it yourself, staying focussed on your own health and your dream. I say this to myself: If it doesn't work after six months I can stop doing it. What is six months if the reward is a new life?

It depends on the goal which you want to achieve. I just wanted to lose weight. With this dietary change you will lose weight for sure. You will also hear about many other options to lose weight.

But consider the following: you, as a sick person, might have different needs to a so-called healthy person. Healthy people often forget that you are ill and they tend to measure according to their own criteria. For example, you are not allowed to lose muscle mass which is inevitable with every type of diet - you need every gram of muscle. So stick to your OWN plan and lose weight in the right way for yourself. If someone else has already reached his goal weight he has to build up muscle too, but in the right way for him. Training suitable for so-called healthy people is not necessarily suitable for us, at least not in the beginning. So don't give up.

05 April 2014: The new diet is delicious. Thank God. Now Petra shares my sentiments and enjoys it too. What I have noticed is that I don't desire meat or sweets anymore.

My dear darling Petra liked the new diet as much as I did and she supported me in every way. There is simply nothing bad about healthy food. What used to be just a side-dish is now a main dish. You can eat as many vegetables and fruit as you like. What could be bad about that? Your partner doesn't have to eat as much as you do, but he/she needs to support you with your plans and try to avoid speaking against it. You will recognise that your sense of taste will change too. Due to food enhancements and additives from industries, your sense of taste has already been changed and now with the absence of these chemical additives, everything changes again.

I only can say that everything tastes delicious and I don't have to have sweets because Mother Nature has provided me with enough sweetness in fruit. No one needs to cook an extra meal for you - they need only prepare more of the salad.

In addition, there is nothing wrong with trying out new things and relinquishing meat or instant meals a couple of times a week. Understandably, everyone should be satisfied and happy with his meal - there is nothing worse than having to starve, or having to eat something you don't like.

17 April 2014: I started to take vitamin D3 and K2 in large doses. 100.000 IE D3 per day, and 10 pieces of K2 equally portioned, three times a day. I observe my body very accurately and try to write down how I feel, and any possible changes. I expect nothing but every day I hope to get a bit better. I don't care if takes a long time, but each day I wish for a little miracle to happen. It's ok to wish for something. 104 kg!

Regrettably I didn't start this treatment earlier. I didn't know about it. No doctor advises you about such options. Doctors have been taught that vitamin D3 is dangerous and won't recommend it. I, as an ill person, would like to get heathy and so I look for information in a variety of reliable sources. If one starts to experiment with oneself one needs instructions. Without these it is either dangerous or crazy. I wouldn't suggest you try something without a plan, and without having informed yourself fully about the risks and possible consequences. Like I said, there are a lot of good books which I can highly recommend you read, and only then to go for it and try it out. You don't have to be afraid of small experiments -even a doctor does the same in principle. I am like most people: very impatient when it comes to achieving my goal. On the other hand I have learned to wait.

19 April 2014: My stomach went crazy again. I felt powerless, I was exhausted and my circulation was bad. Obviously I didn't eat enough. I often forget to eat until I feel nauseous. I have to get this under control otherwise I am not able to experience my body in the right way. I am curious about the first changes.

Unfortunately I have consistent problems with my stomach. The lack of muscle affects my whole wellbeing in a negative way. One also has to reckon with recurring setbacks. In contrast to a healthy body, a weak body needs more time to recover. Those recurrent setbacks were a heavy blow for me. One day something is pretty easy to do and the next day the same thing is almost impossible. One has to learn to deal with that fact. If one has 99 bad days out of 100 like me, one gets used to feeling bad all the time. If there is suddenly a series of good days one might well become confused. What was easy yesterday might not be possible today. It's just like that. Be glad to experience ever more good days in between. These good days will get more numerous. Enjoy them!

23 April 2014: Today we fetched wheels from Petras garage. Also we took the new slats for our bed with us. After the whole trip I still have a lot of energy left. From where, I don't know. I haven't got more strength, but a lot more energy. I'll have to watch how I feel tomorrow. Even recovering after being exhausted happened faster. After only two hours of lying down I was able to walk a couple of steps again. I am excited about today's accomplishment. Even Yoga was easier than normal. Today I took 20 mg Lioresal less.

That was a 'wow-day'. Getting up in the morning I noticed that I was full of energy. I described it like this: "It feels as if someone has switched the light on in me." The strange thing was that I didn't have more power, but the energy came back into my body like a rocket. I was full of beans and simply had to do something about it. We were active the whole day and I didn't get tired. I was totally puzzled and thought: "Is that already the effect of the vitamin D3 drops?" Yes, it was. And still to this day those drops haven't lost their effect.

But I also had to come to terms with the fact that I didn't actually gain any strength. I was full of energy and desperate to get out of my flat, but I didn't have enough power to walk. It was extremely annoying, but I had to learn how things worked and accept that regaining my strength would only happen bit by bit, and take much longer. It improved a little, day by day. But what was very important and showed that I had made a step in the right direction, was that I got my missing energy back. On this day I decided to reduce the Lioresal remedy. In any case I was taking too much of it.

25 April 2014: Walking is difficult today and once again I am out of energy. I am tired and my legs feel like lead! They feel as if I have pins and needles and there is an irritating 'stretching' feeling in my shins. I notice that my right hand has got warmer although it stings from time to time. Up to now it was always cold. No sensitivity, no movement possible. Lying down helps only a little. I remain tired and listless. That annoying eczema behind my ear has improved. I just happened to notice it today; I have had it for a long time, treating it with Cortisone for over a year without success. I must watch how it develops further.

As it turned out, after the first energy-loaded day I was so knackered that I needed two days off to recover. However the D3 drops started to be effective. I had new sensations in my body such as the sudden appearance of pins and needles in my legs and the stretching in the shin bones. Although I still felt listless I could no longer ignore a certain 'stirring-up' starting in my body. What impressed me most of all was the warming of my hand.

26 April 2014: For the first time in years, when I got up this morning I had almost no spasms and cramps (80% less). I felt a burning and pulling from my instep to the shinbone and up to my right knee. My hand stayed warm although it remained, as always, numb and stiff. The pain in my joints from permanently lying down has reduced to 90%. I can feel certain movements now, but without pain. Altogether I feel softer, more flexible, more relaxed and liberated from old pains. Admittedly there are new unpleasant feelings in my legs and hand, but they seem different. Today I won't take any medicine. Let's see what the night may bring.

Almost all spasms and cramps stopped. I couldn't believe it. For years I had suffered from them but now they had almost disappeared. I didn't have any further pains. It happened overnight and I could hardly believe it. I thought to myself, this would be how someone on drugs might feel. Just nine days had passed and so much has happened to me. I was really euphoric, but at the same time frightened that it may not last. As I said, with these ups and downs came various psychological challenges. And then, in my over- eagerness I made a mistake.

27 April 2014: The night was horrible. I couldn't sleep and eventually gave in and took a pill at 2 am. To cut medication out altogether wasn't a good idea at all. What was I thinking? I have strong pain in my left shoulder, slight pain in the right shoulder. Because of the pain I couldn't sleep until 5 am. At noon we drove to the Danube and enjoyed the warm sun. Good feeling in my legs but no power today. I am constantly at my limits and have to lie down. Hand warm. Body moving without pain. I am able to lift my arm up to my shoulder. The hand is still warm but numb and stiff. The incredible progress of the last days is fantastic. Strength and walking not much better, am constantly exhausted and tired. Evening: I am feeling soft and flexible. I fell down and was able to crawl on hands and legs. I can crawl very awkwardly, but previously, due to a lack of strength and energy I was not even able to do that. When I pee it burns a little as if I would have sand in my bladder.

Leaving the medication out was a mistake. I strongly advise against stopping all medication all at once. The bill came immediately in the form of pain. What does one do when one cannot sleep because of the pain? One can suffer or, like I did, do mental arithmetic. One can also locate the pain and try to speak inwardly to it. Then I ask: "What do you want? Why are you there?" The pain does not come for nothing. Your body speaks to you. You only have to learn to listen to it. I didn't always listen to it and each time I got a heavy bill for it. That's the good thing about our bodies – they always tell us immediately what they are uneasy about. (Is that why in English it's called a dis-ease?).

30 April 2014: In the morning slight spasms and cramps again. At 10 am when I had to pee a kidney stone passed without pain! Now I know why nothing changed in the last days: my body needed its power and concentration for the kidney stone. I had no renal colic like before and no pain. Now I am curious about any possible changes in my body now that the stone has passed. Movement, the ability to walk, endurance and strength have to improve.

Over the years, from time to time, I have had problems with renal colic and kidney stones. The first thing a body does when it goes into healing mode is purge all the important organs that clean and detox the body. As the stones passed my kidneys could start to function fully again. The good thing about it this time is that it happened without the dreaded renal colic. While the body is in healing mode it needs to concentrate on one area and possibly take energy from other organs. One feels drowsy, listless, fatigued. The goings-on in the 'background' are not noticed until they are done. That's the reason why one has to sleep so much when one is ill. That's all there is to it. So do not become desperate, just wait and see.

05 Mai 2014: Getting up this morning I was able to move the big toe on my right leg. I haven't been able to do that for years. The shin bone nerve, which controls the toes, has been paralyzed since 2008. I can't believe it; I am excited like a little child. Yippee. At noon I was still able to move my toe. With help from Petra I could walk 100 m at the Danube. I was extremely tired after the walk and had to go home immediately to sleep. Heels, calves, thighs tingle a lot. Today I took 20mg less of the Lioresal again. Hydal 16 mg.

New things are happening constantly. An exciting time. Walking gets easier and easier. Slowly my persistence is paying off. I was always tired after my walks but at the same time very glad to be able to do the distance. The gradual reduction of medication seems to be the right way.

15 May 2014: I have established a new training program. I do Yoga for 15-20 minutes every day. Unfortunately I only started doing Yoga on a daily basis now. I should have started it years ago. At noon went shopping. I am totally amazed at how much strength and endurance I have today. 15 minutes of shopping and walking to the car. After that, homewards and into bed as I was totally exhausted. But it was a good feeling to have been active for so long.

I would recommend Yoga to everyone, even though it might be difficult in the beginning. Every kind of meditation, Yoga or Tai-Chi is valuable. Most important is the regularity. Sadly I didn't always do it this way. I can certainly understand anyone who says they are too tired or feeling too ill. But do try to practice even if for only 5 minutes. It will help you a lot in the long run. Over and over again I was amazed by my achievements in Yoga or Tai-Chi. Even just the concentrated standing and slow movements can lead to 'Aha-experiences' every now and again. And afterwards you will realise that there is a lot more within you than you might have thought.

18 May 2014: I am very weak and tired. Walking is not possible as I am just too weak. I was very tired yesterday and went to bed at 11:15 pm.

Today I lay in bed until 10:30 am because I was still tired. 15:25 pm another kidney stone passed without pain. Now I know why I felt so weak yesterday. 100 kg!!!

Tiredness could be an indication that your body is busy dealing with things. Trust it. If you treat it in the right way it will do its best. I have lost 10 kg without starving. The kg disappeared on their own just by me eating the right things. And without losing any energy. Actually just the opposite happened - I gained energy.

22 May 2014: Bad night's sleep. My right kidney is a bit sensitive but it doesn't hurt too much. In the garage of the shopping mall I had a very emotional experience: pushing the shopping cart I was able to move my right leg in such a way that I could almost walk normally for about 5 m! I nearly cried with happiness.

Everyone who is willing to work on himself will have such experiences. Out of nothing my leg moved naturally. The body seems to have a capacity for remembering. And when the time is right it recalls it. Unfortunately I only managed to walk a few steps like that and later that same day I wasn't able to repeat it at all. There is a difference between being an adult and being a baby: a baby has to learn everything new, but your adult body knows how to organise itself and is thus able to learn faster. It remembers everything it was previously able to do.

Thinking back to my first moving on the floor; there was not much difference compared to a baby. Everything is difficult or partly impossible. This period of change brought some very painful and difficult situations with it.

My body's posture changed. Ligaments, sinews and muscles had to adapt. The aches can be pretty severe and last for weeks. I always had problems with my sciatic nerve and now I notice aches and pains in exactly this area of my body. Although now they feel quite different: they are there because of all the new movements, such as my uprightness and walking.

29 May 2014: Slept well. I am very relaxed this morning. I even slept on my right side. I had the need to lie on my right side and for the first time in years I did it without pain! Getting out of bed was super easy. I am full of energy. Again I took 20 mg less Lioresal. Hydal 8 mg.

The movements and posture of my body are strange to me because I had become used to moving differently. I woke up lying on the right side of my body and I couldn't believe it - nothing hurt; I was able to lie like that for over an hour. A lot of things happen during the night.

31 May 2014: Slept well. I was able to lie on my right side for over 5 hours without problems and significantly fewer spasms and cramps. Walking and standing straight after getting up is more difficult than normal as I need time to loosen up. The body has to wake up properly first. The whole right arm is very warm, lifting and moving is easy but hand and fingers are still stiff. Sense of balance is weak today. Body generally feeling worse than other days.

During this period the life came back slowly to my right arm. Physically, I experienced ups and downs each day. Something odd occurred: straight after getting up this morning I had to lie down again and after going to the toilet I was totally exhausted. I didn't actually fall asleep but my body needed about an hour to wake up.

06 June 2014: Energy and body feeling good. Today I lay in the sun at the Danube. I lay on the hard ground without any pain. Despite a full 20 minutes of sunshine I was not over hot. I am coping ever better with warmth and sunshine. The light seems to be rather good for me. Although I do notice that too much heat over the day stresses my body if I don't cool down now and again. I fell and needed help to get up. Right hand feels better, not so extremely numb, it's warm but swollen.

During the summers I always had air conditioning at home to make things more bearable. Heat is generally more difficult for someone with MS. My limit was around 73°F – 77°F and anything over that made my condition worse; I was hardly able to move and everything was more of a challenge than normal. But now I was coping much better with the heat and was even able to go out into the sun. We drove to a wonderful place directly on the Danube where I could sun myself and practice walking.

09 June 2014: Today I walked 100 m alone with my walking stick at the Danube. Petra didn't help me. My leg dragged on the ground but generally it felt good walking. I got into a cramp, probably because I wasn't used to walking alone and free, and also because I was afraid of falling. Today I was able to get up from the floor all alone for the first time after Yoga! But I needed a chair or a table as support - I have to hold on to something.

The results of training and exercising became noticeable. I was able to walk alone for longer distances. At the beginning I cramped totally and thus my gait pattern became worse. But I didn't give up and every day I fought for every inch.

The fear of falling and getting hurt was at the back of my mind the whole time. For my own safety Petra was permanently at my side. Just knowing that someone is by your side, and how lucky you are to have someone on whom you can rely and who is with you the whole time, is very helpful indeed.

19 June 2014: I am feeling good and fresh. Went walking at the Danube again. With Petra we walked a straight 250 m! My hand isn't so stiff in the evening. Fingers start to move slowly. 98 kg!

Set yourself big goals every day. But set them so that they are also realistic, achievable.

21 June 2014: Again at the Danube. I walked 300 m with Petras help! Afterwards I was wiped out and my back hurt badly. My posture is getting better and the distance was a new record for me! My hand is slowly improving. The results of training on a daily base are noticeable. Sadly the feeling in my hand is not improving - I am able to grasp something but I am not able to feel it. Hydal 4 mg.

Sometimes, after these (for me very long) walking exercises, I was so wiped out that I would sit or lie down for long periods at the Danube. During this time I would read a lot and learn how the body functions.

29 June 2014: Today I took 20 mg less Lioresal. Went 200 m with my walking stick, but alone! Balancing exercises with the guide ropes in my living room become easier.

For me, the little records were the highlight of each day. I was so excited about regaining my quality of life step by step each day. I have guide ropes hanging from the ceilings of my flat as I always need something to hold on to whilst moving. I also use these chords for my training sessions.

13 July 2014: Was at the Danube again and with Petra and walked 500 m straight. After that I was physically exhausted, but not tired. Right leg was very weak afterwards. Sitting to rest is less helpful for regeneration. I have to lie down, need two hours to recover. Today I didn't take any Hydal. I have to see what happens.

When I overdo things such as when walking or exercising I have to lie down and I don't care where. For that reason I always have a deck chair in my car. I can also lie down in my car.

16 July 2014: Today I got my new bar-bells and began to practice immediately. The right hand is able to hold the 1.5 kg, even though I can't feel it. I do exercises for the strengthening of my wrists and for a good grip. 96 kg!

When I noticed my strength increasing I borrowed bar-bells from friends with changeable weights. I started with 1.5 kg. In the beginning it was hard work for me. I held the 1.5 kg weight in my hand until it dropped. I stood next to my couch so that the bar-bell would not make a noise by dropping onto the floor. Each day a couple of seconds more, that was my target.

21 July 2016: Today at 10 pm I only took 10 mg Lioresal. I have reduced it from 100 – 125 mg daily to 10 mg and I am feeling good.

The slow reduction of medicine was an important step in the right direction. Every medicine you introduce into your body has to be removed. The release pays off in the long run. You will soon recognise when you are ready to reduce something, and how your body may react to that change. Just don't go too fast. Everything takes time. Have faith in your own body. If you don't disturb it, it will do the right thing. Forget about your ego and let your body act. You will be surprised at what it is able to do.

04 August 2014: Today during my bar-bell training I had a strong hold until the end. My joints are getting stronger and stronger. I was able to walk 500 m alone with my stick. After that I was totally wiped out and needed one hour to recover until finally I was able to drive home.

Everything has its own time. Just take the time you need. When I managed to walk 500m alone I knew that I had regained a big part of my independence. 500 m is far enough that I can walk anywhere I may need to go on my own. I just have to take care and not fall, which unfortunately I still do from time to time. During this period I did biceps and triceps exercises, because everything has atrophied over the years.

11 August 2014: Was able to stand for a whole hour. Afterwards I was very tired but not completely wiped out like before. In Yoga for the first time I was able to stand alone for a standing exercise without holding onto something.

I constantly practiced standing alone to overcome the side-effects and complications due to a weak sense of balance.

When I think back on how I used to be able to only stand for one or two minutes, I am very proud of my achievements. Yes, you are allowed to be proud of yourself and your achievements. Forget what they taught you. You are allowed; in fact you should actively praise yourself.

With Yoga one exercises the sense of balance too. I have huge problems with balance and I have had to fight for every second to be able to stand freely again. Closing my eyes during standing was impossible as I would have fallen over immediately. I needed two chairs to hold on to for Yoga. Today the trend was broken and I was able to stand completely free during an exercise. For me there is a difference between standing upright and stationary, and moving while in a standing position. Standing and moving was not as bad as I could somehow compensate my imbalance.

13 August 2014: Went walking at the Danube and after 150 m I fell and bruised my ribs and my hip and right hand. Knee and elbow were grazed and cut on broken rocks. Could not get up alone and Petra had to help me. In the evening my whole right side and right hand hurt. Tried to ease the pain with Yoga but it was damn painful! I had fallen often enough but had never hurt myself quite this bad. This time I fell stupidly.

I can remember it very clearly. I was overzealous and didn't take care, wanting to increase my pace. Then it happened. I fell, and in that moment I knew that I had hurt myself more than the other times. I couldn't breathe and my right wrist and ribs hurt badly. I could not do a thing about it and Petra had to help me up. We went back to the car and I sat down to catch my breath.

After that we drove home so I could lie down. I noticed that I was in mild shock.

I had to get a grip on the fear rising up in me. It is very important not to go walking alone. I never did walk alone. If you fall and hurt yourself you may not be able to help yourself at all. This helplessness can create psychological problems. Fear itself can paralyze you, and then you may not manage to walk at all. Without support I wouldn't have been able to walk all the way back to the car.

17 August 2014: Sleep was good but short. Ribs on the right still hurt but a lot better than yesterday. Went two rounds in the hall today: 108 steps up und 108 steps down = 216 steps + 300 m to walk. On the second round it was very difficult to walk. After Yoga right side of my ribs hurts. Again a bad sense of balance.

I trained a lot and became stronger and stronger and could endure more. Unfortunately my sense of balance has not improved much, otherwise I would do more.

19 August 2014: A walk around the house. During the day very tired again. Slept for an hour in the afternoon. From today no more Lioresal. As from today I am free of medication!

That was a memorable day for me. After years of taking medicine I was completely free of it for the first time!

16 September 2014: Right hand is very warm and I can move my fingers. The life has come back to my hand.

Am able to grasp things, have some strength, and even a bit of feeling in my palm. Very little, but it is alive again!

That was the beginning of an up-and-down road with my right hand. This initial sense of feeling in my palm disappeared later, but returned every now and again thereafter.

06 October 2014: Today a kidney stone passed without pain. In the last two weeks I have only a slight burning or stinging when urinating, but no pain. No colic. The body detoxes itself.

That was not the last kidney stone in 2014.

27 November 2014: A very tiny kidney stone passed at noon. No pain.
And that was still not the last one.

02 December 2014: Again a kidney stone passed, no pain.

Yes, that's how it works with detoxing. The body reduces the excess uric acid. If detoxing goes too fast then everything combines as a kidney stone. That was the last one in 2014!

25 December 2014: Got strong feeling in my palm and fingers. In the morning I was able to feel almost everything. I am totally amazed. Able to move my fingers and for the first time in years I can feel everything I touch. Indeed not 100 %, but at least I can feel something. Consciously grasping at something is possible even with closed eyes! Yippee!

CHAPTER 14: WHAT HAS CHANGED IN MY LIFE?

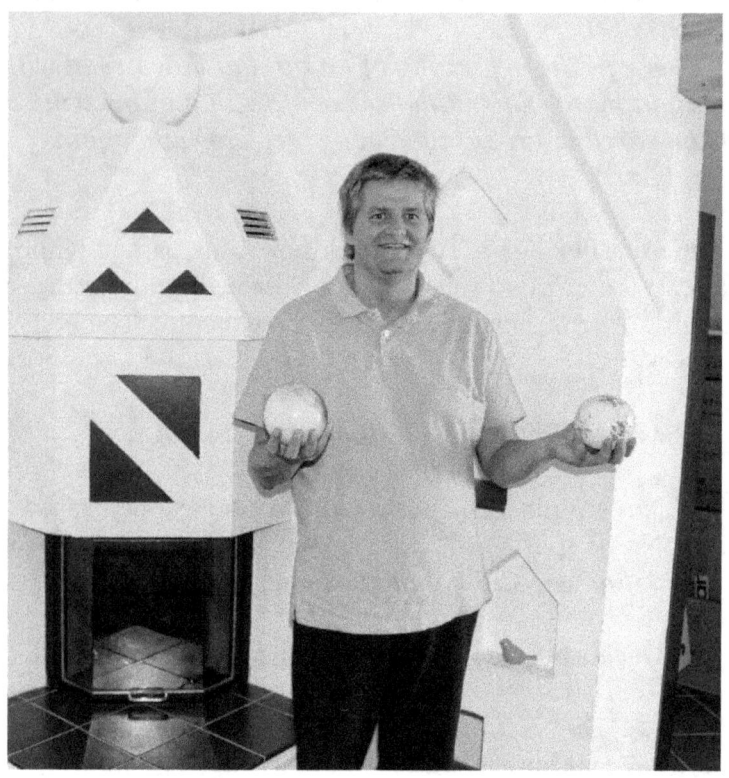

The year was almost over and everybody asked, "What has he changed in his life?"

A lot changed in my life in the year 2014!

- My cramps and spasms have reduced by 99%;
- The fatigue-syndrome has disappeared, as has the pain;
- The psoriasis and eczema have reduced by 95%;
- I am able to sleep for six to eight hours at a stretch and can even lie on my right side;

- I can walk with a walking stick so I am not wheelchair-bound. See *pictures 8A* and *8B* in the gallery;
- The agonising periods of being bedridden and dependent on nursing care are over as I have begun to live a new life;
- I am now helping others who are ill and who had given up because they couldn't find a way out;
- The arthrosis in my knee has improved so much that I don't need a leg splint anymore;
- The paralysis in my right arm and hand has improved and I am now able to grab onto and hold something;
- I have regained my gross motor skills and am now working on my fine motor skills;
- I began to play saxophone again. My playing may be torture for my audience but I don't care. In summer the mosquitos stayed away from my flat;
- The most important change is my growing courage to face life, and my *new joie de vivre*! I have lots to do in the upcoming year and am determined to make further improvements and set and achieve new goals. More of that in my next book.

An Indian proverb:

> **"Everything is good in the end,
> and if it's not, it´s not the end!"**

CHAPTER 15: WHAT ARE THE NEXT STEPS?

My second book: *Masterplan zum Erfolg (Masterplan for Success)*

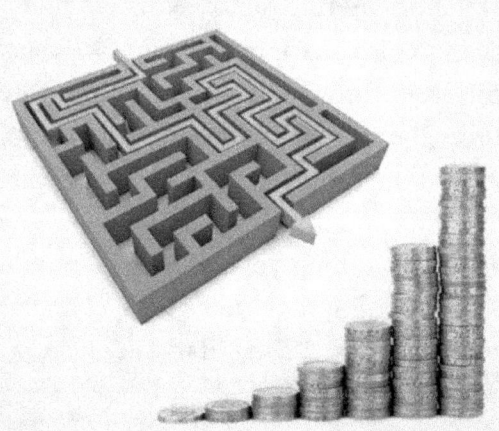

I wrote three more books during 2015 and 2016. My second book, *Masterplan zum Erfolg* (currently available only in German), describes in detail how one can develop the 'RIGHT DREAM' and set the appropriate 'RIGHT TARGETS' for oneself. I describe in detail how to motivate yourself with my '5-S' technique. The '5-S-Strategy' is the most important tool of all. You will learn how to develop the right attitude and a firm belief in YOURSELF. The '5-S-Strategy' was developed in response to several questions and discussions with people attending my lectures. I recognised that most people lacked one thing: A masterplan!

Chapter overview
Chapter 1 – Instruction manual for the workbook
Chapter 2 – Discover your potential
Chapter 3 – Find your dream
Chapter 4 – How to reach a goal
Chapter 5 – We can only be successful through others; what is success for you?
Chapter 6 – Childhood traumas and anti- success programs
Chapter 7 – Stress, perfectionism and burnout
Chapter 8 – Anti anger program
Chapter 9 – Positive thinking
Chapter 10 – Motivation
Chapter 11 – The '5-S-Strategy'
Chapter 12 – Courage and anxiety
Chapter 13 – Shame and death - a taboo
Chapter 14 – Joy and sadness
Chapter 15 – How our economy works

My third book: *Angst im Kopf (A Psyche of Fear)*

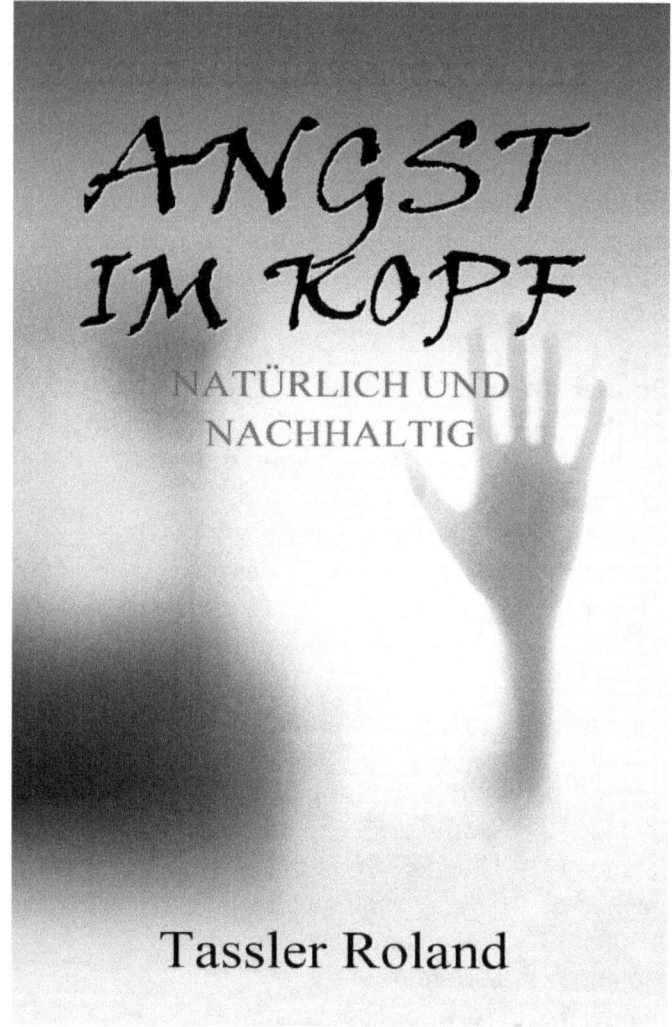

My third book, "Angst im Kopf" (currently available only in German) also rose out of observations and conversations with audiences at my lectures.

In my opinion it is the most important issue of all. Most people fail only because of their fears, not daring to make a change. Anxiety, shame and fear are the biggest killers of success. In this book I explain how anxiety can paralyze us and how everybody is able to overcome it.

Chapter overview
Chapter 1 - Anxiety
Chapter 2 - Fear
Chapter 3 - Shame
Chapter 4 – Anxiety for living
Chapter 5 – Fear of death
Chapter 6 – Overcoming anxiety

My fourth book: *Tabu (Taboos)*
(The book is currently available only in German)

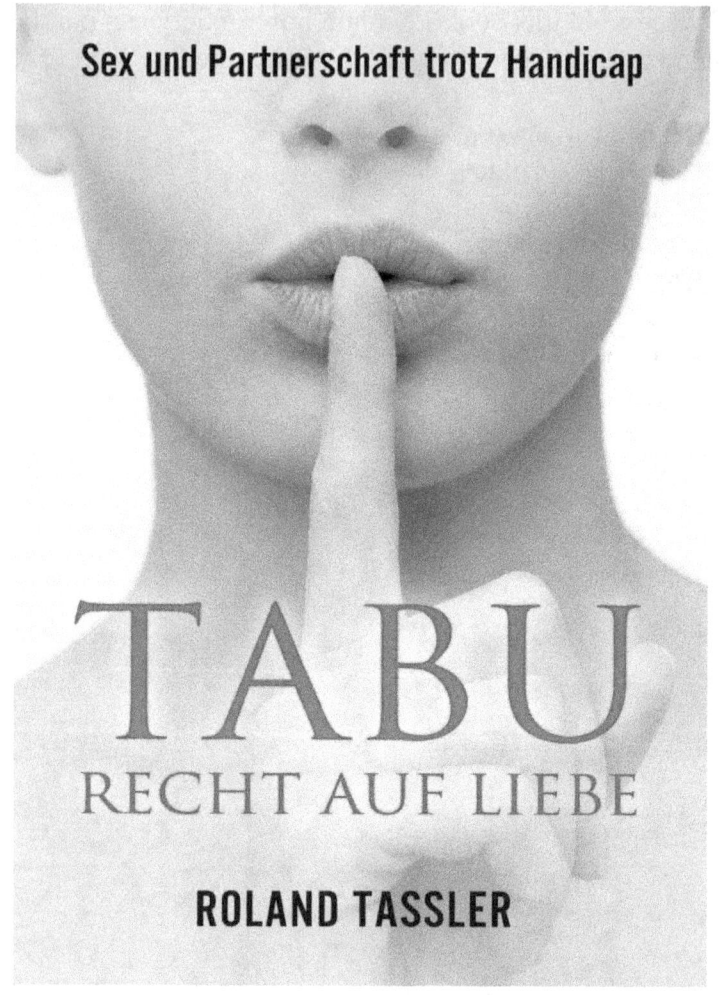

A 'taboo' is something no one wants to talk about. Why should one not be allowed to speak about love, sex and partnerships for disabled people? Is society itself too inhibited or 'unable'?

Whoever claims that disabled or chronically ill persons don't want or need sexuality in their lives is wrong. This book attempts to describe, with ruthless honesty, what affected people think about love, sex and partnership, and how they experience it with all its highs and lows. It is not always easy to live out one's sexuality, but all the more fun and fulfilling when one knows how. That is the focus of this book, which offers many hints and ideas. It also shares the earnest challenges of the healthy person living with a disabled partner.

In addition, *Tabu* offers solutions in your search for a partner with your own **REVOLUTIONARY PARTNER FORMULA**, which reveals how many potential partners are out there for you. **This 'partner formula' is new** and applicable for everyone! It offers new perspectives on identifying a suitable partner. I share a lot of experience in this area having gone through it all myself. You will recognise that there is a partner out there who is just waiting for you. Yes, indeed.
This book can change your life!

Chapter overview
Chapter 1 – Disabled and single
Chapter 2 – Where and how I can find the right partner?
Chapter 3 - Living with a disabled person
Chapter 4 – Taboo subject: sexuality
Chapter 5 – Disabled yet successful
Chapter 6 – My belief in God and the creation
Chapter 7 – What is going to happen next?

What I do today

Currently I am writing my fifth book. (Appearance January 2017) I literally feel driven to share my knowledge and successes with as many people as possible. I hope I am able to help others like me in one or another constructive way to overcome anxiety, reservations and wrong, externally-controlled doctrines, and to motivate everyone on a steady journey towards being successful, healthy and happy, and to finding their true self, their true 'I'.

I am regularly invited to give lectures where I happily share my knowledge and experiences. If you would like to organise a lecture for people in your surrounds I would be very glad to hear from you.

If you know anyone who would benefit from one of my books, please don't hesitate to recommend me.

I, for myself, will continue on my road of progress and help others wherever I can. So many wonderful things have happened in my life to enable me to get back a life that was denied me for many years. And for that I am extremely grateful and would like to share it.

Don't hesitate to join my website, www.masterplanzumerfolg.com, and stay up to date.

With deepest sincerity I wish you all the best with your efforts, and hope that you will find your own path, and that you build your strength to walk it unflinchingly.

Best regards,
Roland Tassler

My fourth book: Mein Freund Gott (My friend god)

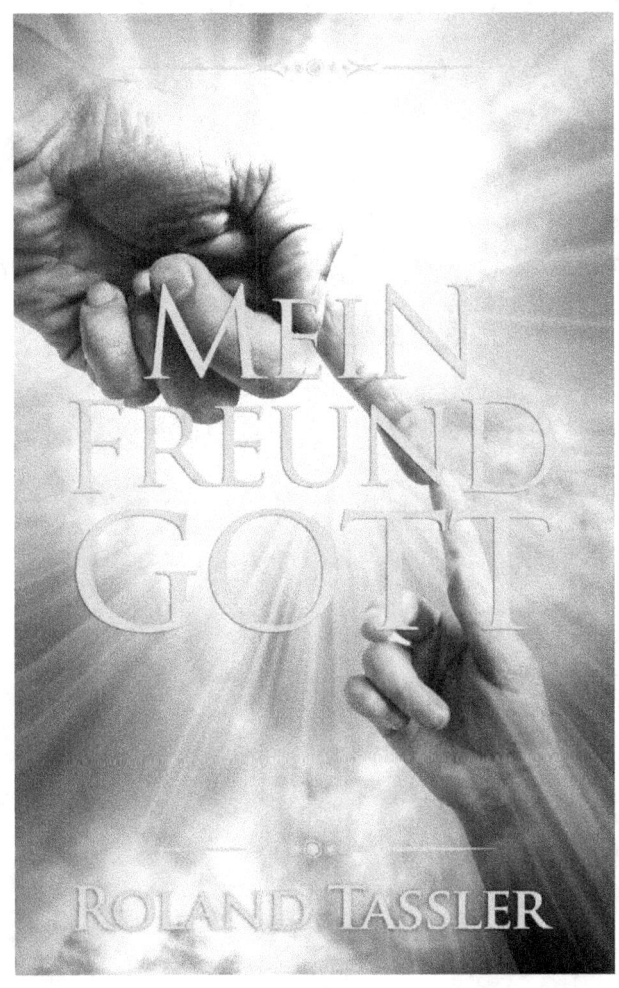

Where to find me

Webpage: www.masterplanzumerfolg.com

Facebook:
https://www.facebook.com/rolandtasslermasterplanzumerfolg/

Email: roland@masterplanzumerfolg.com

Location: Vienna, Austria

PHOTO GALLERY

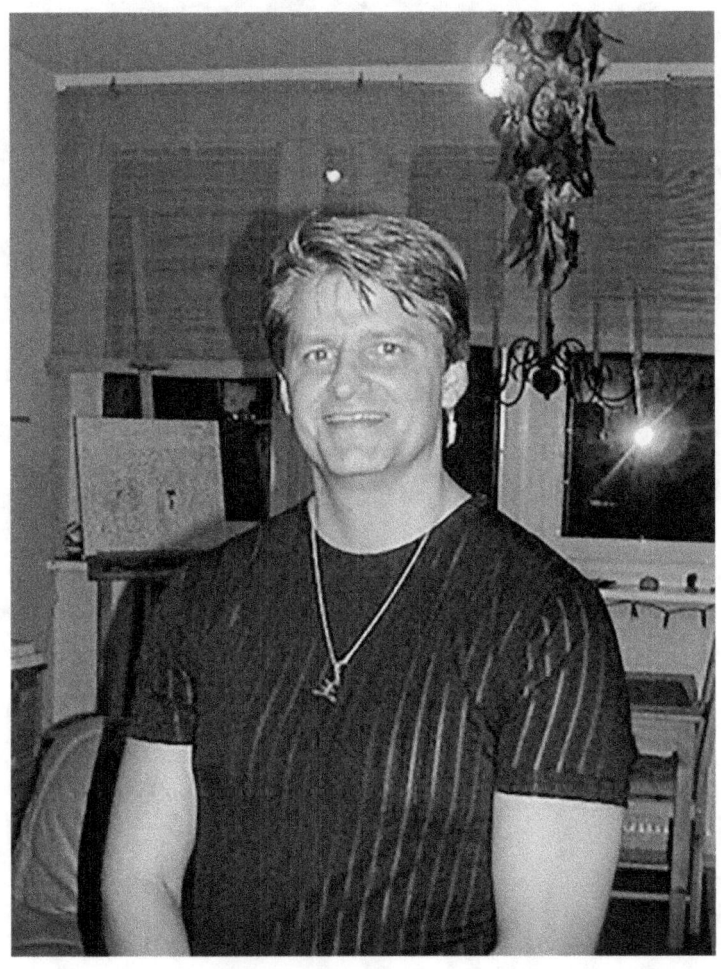

Picture 1: My first life as a young, healthy man

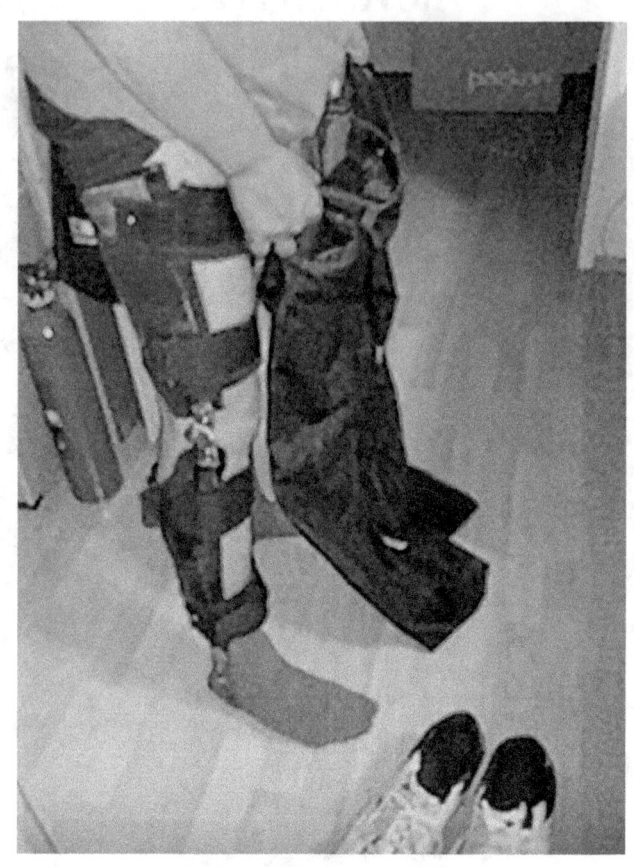

Picture 2: Leg splints

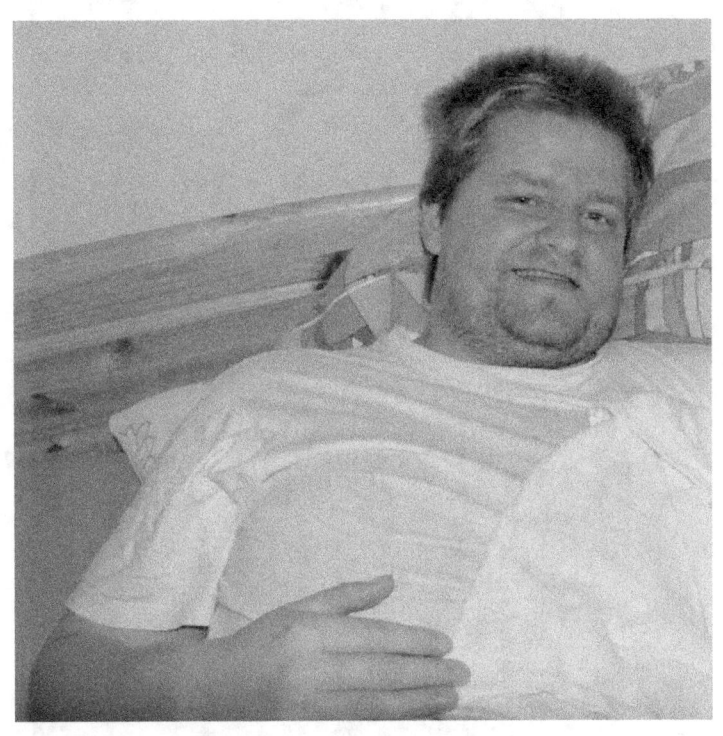

Picture 3: Conscious weight gain

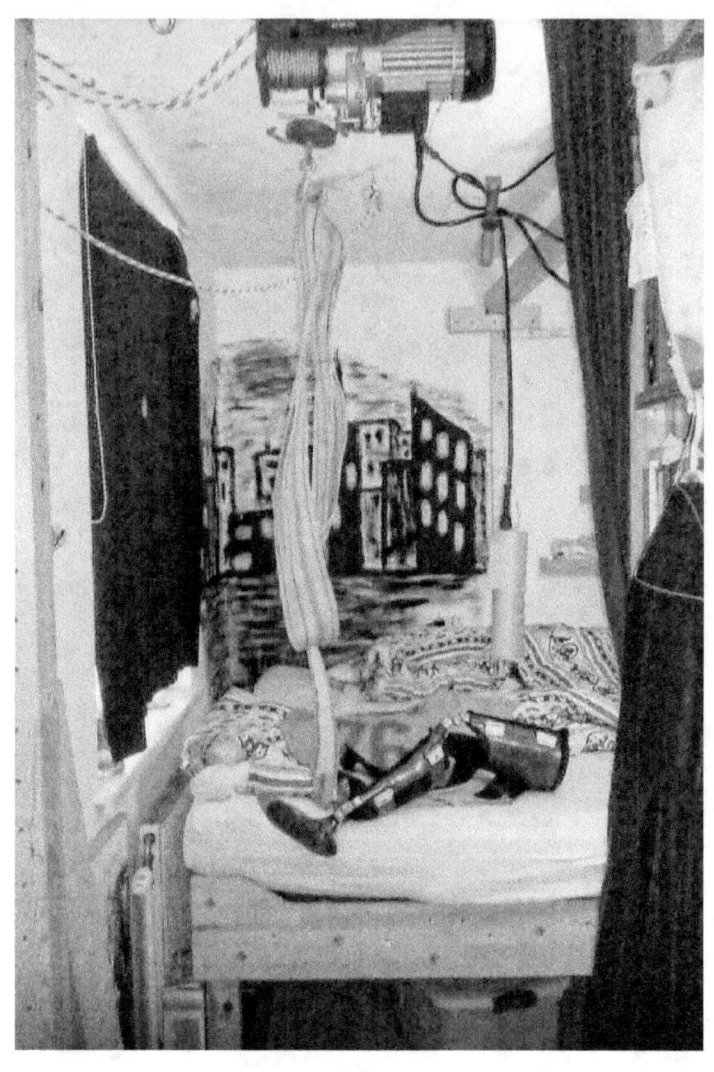

Picture 4A: My bed with ceiling cable crane and leg splints

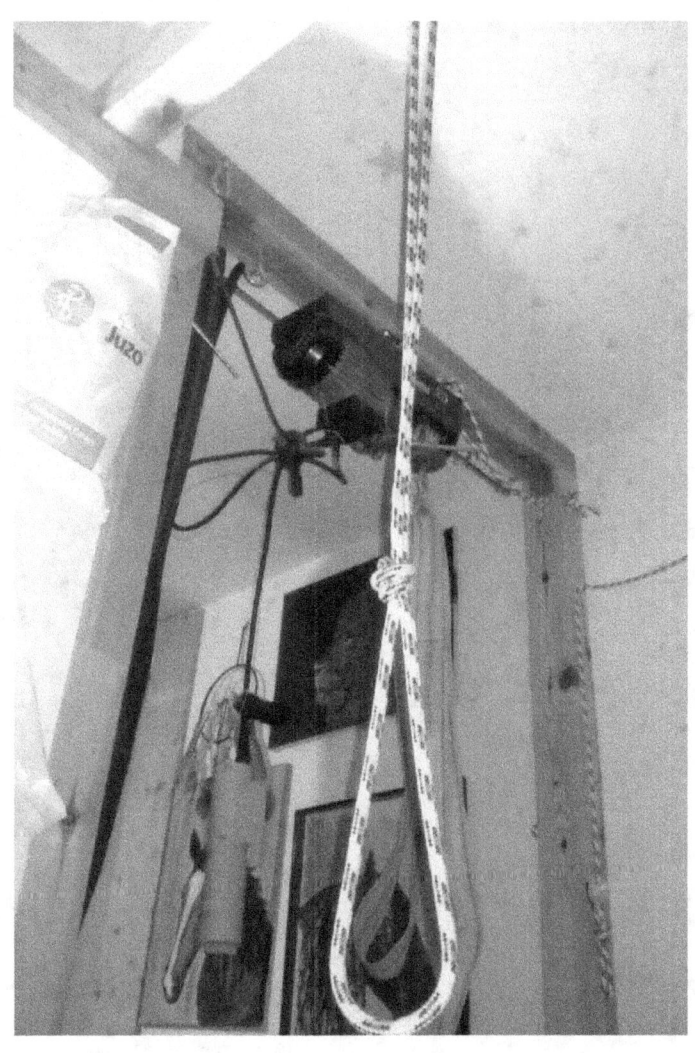

**Picture 4B: Ceiling cable crane and donning loop as
help to move**

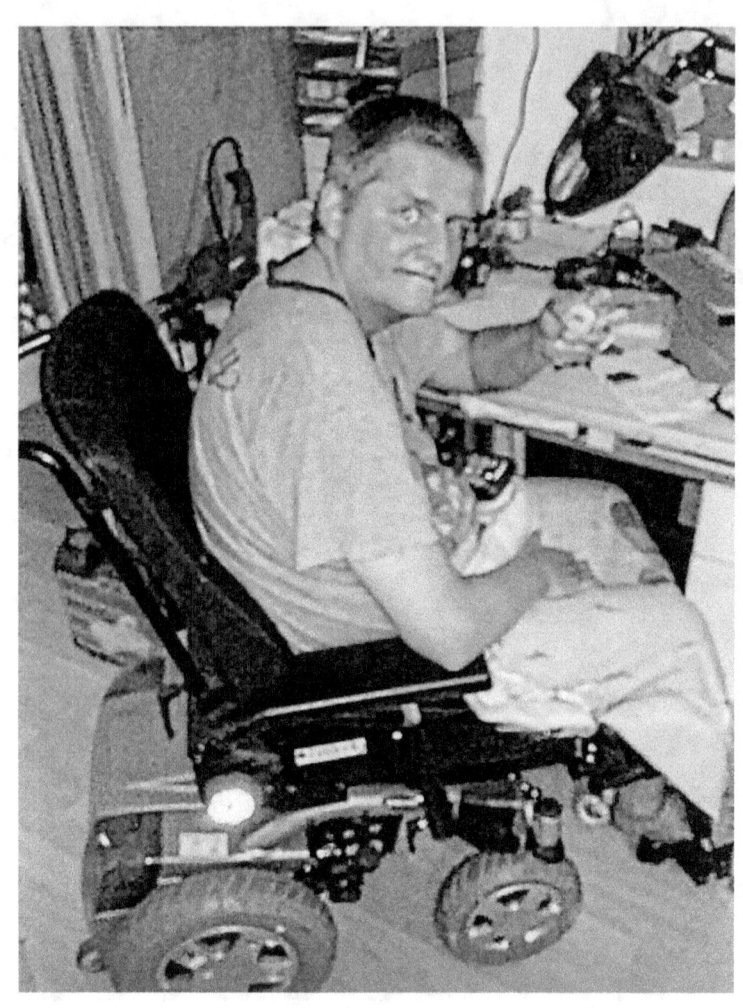

Picture 5: My wagon (wheelchair)

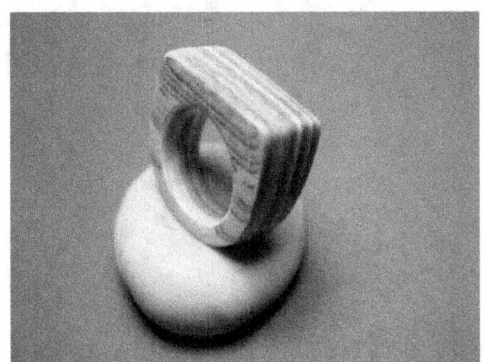

Picture 6: My DIY paper art rings

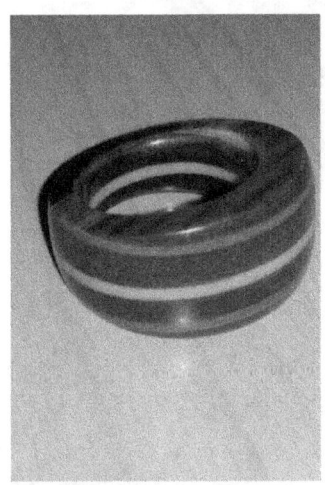

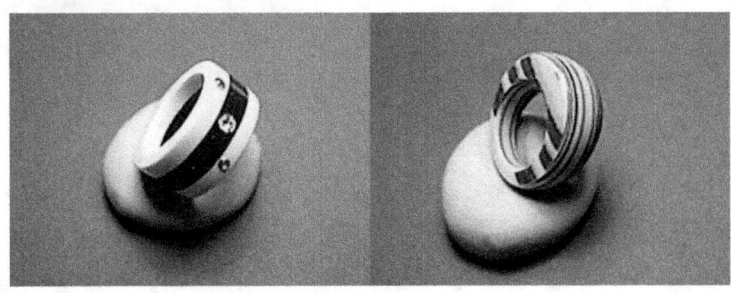

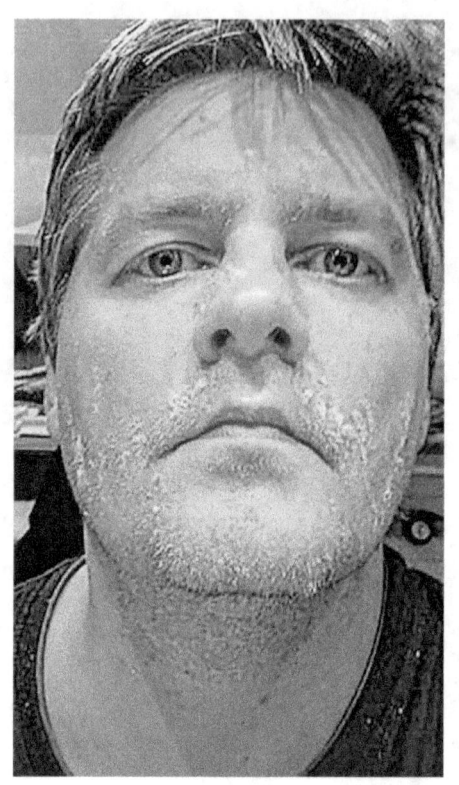

Picture 7: Psoriasis

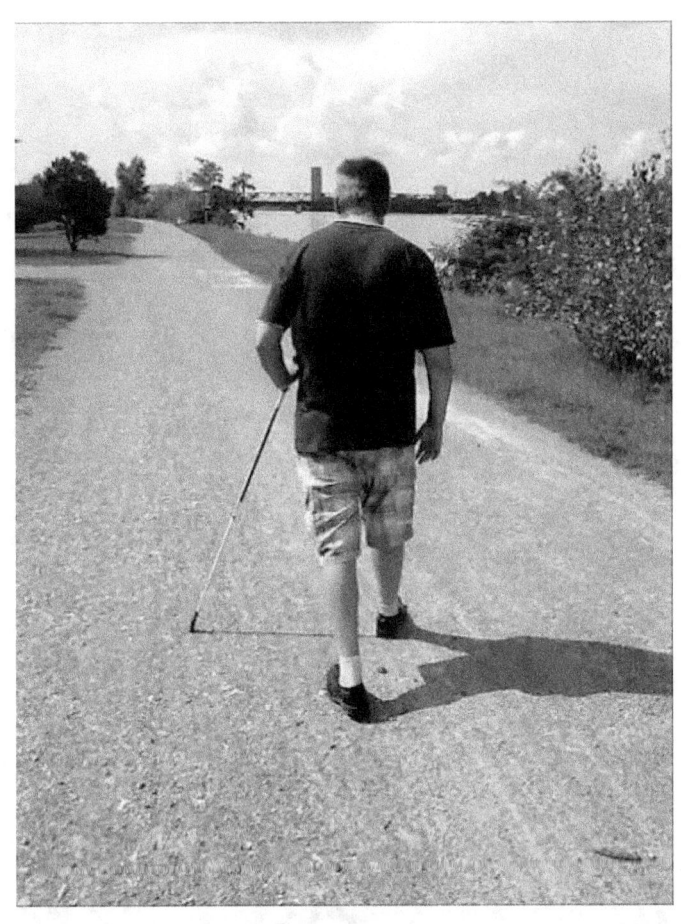

Picture 8A: Walking training at the Danube, slowly but surely…

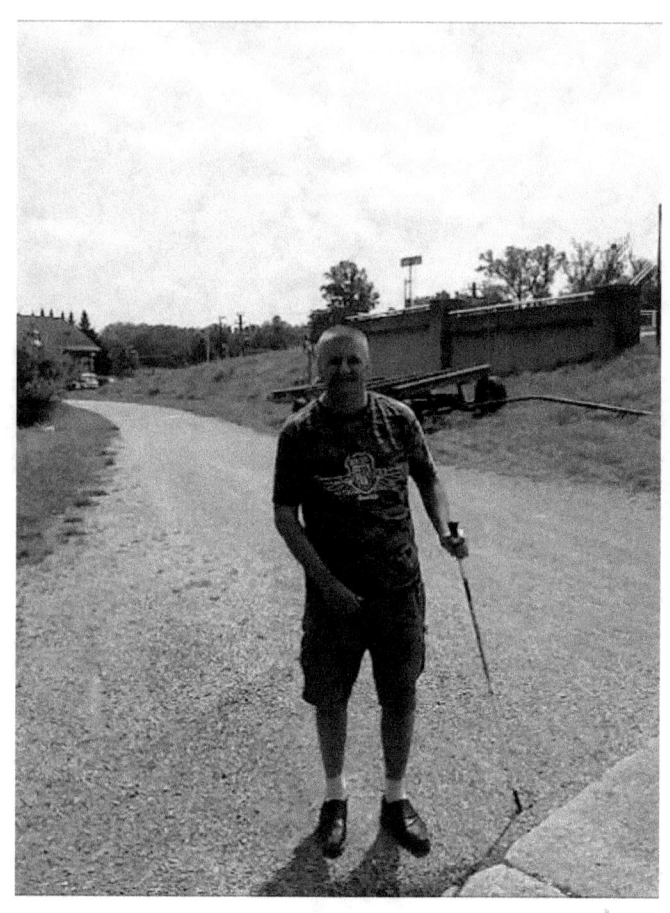

Picture 8B: Walking training at the Danube, ever further…

BONUS RESOURCES

http://masterplanzumerfolg.com/bonus1/

Thank you for buying this book. As a bonus for my readers I have arranged the following links as additional resources. I hope they will help you on your way. I would be happy for any constructive comments, suggestions and questions. I will answer these in prospective blog articles or further books as applicable.

Some selected bonus resources (changes reserved)
- Helpful internet links
- Must-read booklist for everyone, especially for MS-sick people
- Work sheet and instructions, '*Your dream and the goals within*' out of my success program
- Roland Tassler's daily routine
- Various on-site bonus videos from locations described in the book – only for readers of my books
- Other resources as per ongoing requests and demands

FOOTNOTES

[1] Compound Tecfidera: 'Greedy pharma company: This is how it rips off critically ill people', 30 April 2013, from Dani Müller and Christian Schürer, extract: 'Coincidentally scientists discovered that a well-tried active component against Psoriasis is also helpful for someone suffering from the critical illness Multiple Sclerosis. The US-company Biogen exploited this fact and charged thousands of francs for a new medication with an old well-tried component.' (Extract in German only)
http://www.srf.ch/konsum/themen/gesundheit/gierige-pharmafirma-so-zockt-sie-schwerkranke-ab

[2] Wikipedia: Multiple Sclerosis defined
https://en.wikipedia.org/wiki/Multiple_sclerosis

[3] The legend of the Damocles sword
https://en.wikipedia.org/wiki/Damocles

[4] Excerpt from science magazine *scinexx.de* about MS therapy with the active compound Interferon-Beta (Excerpt only in German):
http://www.scinexx.de/wissen-aktuell-17563-2014-05-16.html

[5] Source: Pressetext.com, 'Diagnosis: Death from medication side effects' (Excerpt only in German):
http://www.pressetext.com/news/19980417015

[6] Quotation adapted from Johan Wolfgang von Goethe, Faust I, (2038 f.) The original excerpt is as follows: 'Grey, dear friend, is all theory and green is life's golden tree.'
https://en.wikipedia.org/wiki/Faust,_Part_One

[7]   I had Multiple Sclerosis with the progressive form
https://en.wikipedia.org/wiki/Multiple_sclerosis

[8]   To the medication Fampyra, also see Fampridin
https://en.wikipedia.org/wiki/4-Aminopyridine

[9]   Jeremy May, paper art artist
http://littlefly.co.uk/

[10] Book: *The biology of belief: 'Unleashing the Power of Consciousness, Matter & Miracle*, Bruce Lipton, PhD.
https://www.amazon.de/Biology-Belief-Unleashing-Consciousness-Miracles/dp/1401923127

[11] Brand name Lioresal medication contains the active component Baclofen
https://en.wikipedia.org/wiki/Baclofen

[12] The medicine Hydal is a very effective opioid with the active component Hydromorphone, which is a painkiller.
https://en.wikipedia.org/wiki/Hydromorphone

[13] Fatigue-Syndrome
https://en.wikipedia.org/wiki/Fatigue_(medical)

[14] DVD by Helmuth Matzner: '*Unsere Rückkehr zur Gesundheit*' ('Our return to health', available only in German)
http://helmuthmatzner.com/

[15] Book: '*The Green Foods Bible – Could Green Plants Hold The Key To Our Survival?*' by David Sandoval
https://www.amazon.com/Green-Foods-Bible-David-Sandoval/dp/1893910466

[16] Book: '*The Miraculous Results Of Extremely High Doses Of The Sunshine Hormone Vitamin D3 My Experiment With Huge Doses Of D3 From 25,000 To 50,000 To 100,00 Iu A Day Over A 1 Year Period*', by Jeff T. Bowles
https://www.amazon.com/Miraculous-Results-Extremely-Sunshine-Experiment/dp/1491243821/ref=la_B00AKI5LJC_1_1?s=books&ie=UTF8&qid=1477992057&sr=1-1

[17] YouTube video about Cicero G Coimbra, MD, from Brazil, who reports cure rates of up to 95% with huge doses of Vitamin D3 used by MS-sick or autoimmune disease- suffering people in March 2014. Video shown in Italian language with English subtitles.
https://www.youtube.com/watch?v=hOfO29rL-gl

[18] Book: '*Healthy in seven days – Success through Vitamin D treatment*', by Raimund von Helden, MD
http://www.vitamindservice.com/node/92

[19] Book: **'Water Cures: Drugs Kill: How Water Cured Incurable Diseases'**, by Fereydoon Batmanghelidj, MD

https://www.amazon.com/Water-Cures-Drugs-Incurable-Diseases/dp/0970245815/ref=asap_bc?ie=UTF8

Dr Batmanghelidj discovered the healing effect of water. As a political prisoner of Islamic revolutionists, he was able to save his life and that of others by treating his fellow prisoners with water in spite of the lack of proper food and medicine. He was able to record his healing successes in writing.

[20] Book: ***'Biotop Mensch – Liebe Deine Darmbakterien – Paradigmenwechsel in der Medizin'*** (Biotope human – Love your enterobacteria – a Paradigm shift in medicine; only available in German) https://www.amazon.de/Biotop-Mensch-Darmbakterien-Paradigmenwechsel-Medizin/dp/B005G86ND4/ref=sr_1_2?s=books&ie=UTF8&qid=1481915526&sr=1-2&keywords=biotop+mensch

[21] Books by **Alice Miller: Alice Miller (1923 – 2010)** was a well-known Swiss author and psychotherapist, who wrote books for lay understanding about parent – child relationships. Her insights might help one to understand oneself better.

Among her many books perhaps this one is the best known: **'Prisoner of childhood – The Drama of the Gifted child and the Search for the True Self'**. You may find a list of her books on Amazon in the author pages. https://www.amazon.com/s/ref=sr_st_relevancerank?keywords=Alice+miller&rh=n%3A283155%2Ck%3AAlice+miller&qid=1477994654&sort=relevancerank

[22]   Albert Einstein discovered the theory of relativity as a natural law representing the equivalence of mass and energy. Thus energy is matter and is therefore not able to disappear.

https://en.wikipedia.org/wiki/Mass%E2%80%93energy_equivalence

ACKNOWLEDGEMENT

As a human being I am truly blessed with real friends who have remained at my side despite my illness. Gabriel (Gabor) and Gabriela (Gabi) are among these friends. They helped me to re- join life again. Without their help I would still be bound to the small radius of my home. In their presence one could only feel comfortable and understood. Both of them exude understanding, respect and appreciation as only rarely found. Thank you dear 'Gabis'! The last 22 years with you were a great time for me and I feel honoured to have been allowed to spend them with you. I am so glad I approached you directly 22 years ago, dear Gabor, and said "I have to get to know you because of your wonderful charisma." As I then also got to know your wife, Gabi, I recognised that you are both outstanding human beings.

The next valuable person in my life is Christine Waschulin. Our conversations over the last twenty years have given me the most valuable input. For me you are both muse and example. Unbeknown to you, you became significantly involved with the history and origination of this book. One can only wish for a friend like you. How wonderful that you came into my life!

Thank you Luise Mayerhofer. Your endurance and tenacity are admirable. I have learned so much through our relationship and I am very grateful for our 27 year-long friendship. You always were, and always will be, someone special to me.

Thank you to my mentor, Helmuth Matzner, for supporting me so generously and for giving me the possibility to ease my illness. You believed in me and you gave me back the power to believe in myself again. Your extensive knowledge helped me to improve myself and to find a new and better path to take. I am able to join in with social life again and my overall quality of life has improved. It is thanks to people like you, that people like me regain hope and the chance at a better life. Please never lose heart, just keep going.

The best comes at the end. Dear Petra, thank you so much for always being by my side even through the worst times. You are not only my life partner, but also my support and security. You are one of those special people who are not afraid to share their life with an ill person. You decided to share your life with me even though I was already showing the signs of my illness. You are my star in the night sky. I am filled with joy that you are here, my darling! Many things can't be expressed with words, but I can hold you close to me.

ABOUT ROLAND TASSLER

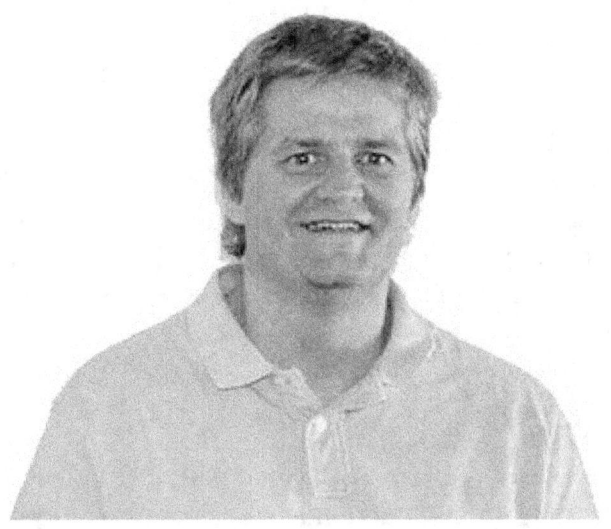

In 2014 I, Roland Tassler, began to order my life in a new way. The autoimmune disease, Multiple Sclerosis, forced me to search for a new path which lead far from conventional medicine. With a lot of courage and self-confidence I was able to improve my condition significantly, which I recorded in my first book, *'My Third Life'*.

My initial condition was **'Hard paralysis, a bedridden case for 24/7 nursing care.'** That 'bodily' element was only one aspect of the whole picture.

What took place in my mind was certainly just as critical. I therefore wrote other books such as *'Masterplan zum Erfolg'* ('Masterplan for success'), *'Angst im Kopf'* ('A psyche of Fear') and *'Tabu'* ('Taboo').

These books (currently available only in German) are suitable for those simply lacking a plan to reach their goals, or to overcome anxieties. After my recovery my main focus was to help others to overcome their own fears of the future.

I took responsibility for my own life and was rewarded with a new 'third life'. Today I am able to walk and stand on my own two feet. I give lectures on this theme and what a person with some will and direction is able to achieve.

I realised that with the right attitude everything is possible. I took the required motivation from the physical successes which I experienced and measured daily. At the same time I never 'unlearned' to dream and constantly set myself new goals to reach.
Through this self-observation and experience I learned to motivate others in similar situations. In my books I share this knowledge of motivation and finding your dream and setting the right goals, and how to find the loopholes in the traps of fear, or the courage to go new successful ways.

You can find more information on my website:
www.masterplanzumerfolg.com
(Website currently only available in German)

IMPRESSUM

Roland Tassler
Rosa Jochmannring 3/15/18
1110 Vienna, Austria
+43 699 1357 2720

roland@masterplanzumerfolg.com
www.masterplanzumerfolg.com

Revised new edition in English

ISBN-13: 978-1541179424

Cover arrangement: Daniel Schenk, Roland Tassler,
Fiverr.com
Cover picture: www.pixbay.com
Other pictures: Roland Tassler, Daniel Schenk
Editing: Daniel Schenk
Translation into English: Bernadine Schneider, Christine
Waschulin

Dependent on the reading device used the text maybe
displayed differently.

www.ingramcontent.com/pod-product-compliance
Lightning Source LLC
Chambersburg PA
CBHW060307290526
45789CB00001B/427